AF213489

Updates on Cardiac Defibrillation, Cardioversion and AED Development

Edited by Endre Zima

Published in London, United Kingdom

Updates on Cardiac Defibrillation, Cardioversion and AED Development
http://dx.doi.org/10.5772/intechopen.105301
Edited by Endre Zima

Contributors
Antonio da Silva Menezes Junior, Thais Aratak Marques Taia, Camila Cássia Canzi, Ana Lígia Valeriano de Oliveira, Lucas Eduardo Almeida França, Aline Lins da Silva, Matheus Araújo Borges, Guilherme Diniz Prudente, Oskars Kalejs, Aija Maca-Kalejs, Ketija Apsite, Anita Abula, Laura Strazdina, Tudor Ovidiu Popa, Diana Cimpoesu, Paul Nedelea, Emilian Manolescu, Alexandra Hauta, Mihaela Corlade-Andrei, Endre Zima, Bettina Nagy, Adam Pal-Jakab, Boldizsar Kiss, Taomin Su, Pan Liu, Qin Shi, Yan Wang, Ying Zhou, Mevlut Demir

© The Editor(s) and the Author(s) 2024

The rights of the editor(s) and the author(s) have been asserted in accordance with the Copyright, Designs and Patents Act 1988. All rights to the book as a whole are reserved by INTECHOPEN LIMITED. The book as a whole (compilation) cannot be reproduced, distributed or used for commercial or non-commercial purposes without INTECHOPEN LIMITED's written permission. Enquiries concerning the use of the book should be directed to INTECHOPEN LIMITED rights and permissions department (permissions@intechopen.com).

Violations are liable to prosecution under the governing Copyright Law.

Individual chapters of this publication are distributed under the terms of the Creative Commons Attribution 3.0 Unported License which permits commercial use, distribution and reproduction of the individual chapters, provided the original author(s) and source publication are appropriately acknowledged. If so indicated, certain images may not be included under the Creative Commons license. In such cases users will need to obtain permission from the license holder to reproduce the material. More details and guidelines concerning content reuse and adaptation can be found at http://www.intechopen.com/copyright-policy.html.

Notice
Statements and opinions expressed in the chapters are these of the individual contributors and not necessarily those of the editors or publisher. No responsibility is accepted for the accuracy of information contained in the published chapters. The publisher assumes no responsibility for any damage or injury to persons or property arising out of the use of any materials, instructions, methods or ideas contained in the book.

First published in London, United Kingdom, 2024 by IntechOpen
IntechOpen is the global imprint of INTECHOPEN LIMITED, registered in England and Wales, registration number: 11086078, 5 Princes Gate Court, London, SW7 2QJ, United Kingdom

British Library Cataloguing-in-Publication Data
A catalogue record for this book is available from the British Library

Additional hard and PDF copies can be obtained from orders@intechopen.com

Updates on Cardiac Defibrillation, Cardioversion and AED Development
Edited by Endre Zima
p. cm.
Print ISBN 978-1-83768-607-0
Online ISBN 978-1-83768-608-7
eBook (PDF) ISBN 978-1-83768-609-4

We are IntechOpen, the world's leading publisher of Open Access books

Built by scientists, for scientists

6,800+
Open access books available

183,000+
International authors and editors

195M+
Downloads

156
Countries delivered to

Our authors are among the
Top 1%
most cited scientists

12.2%
Contributors from top 500 universities

CLARIVATE ANALYTICS BOOK CITATION INDEX INDEXED

WEB OF SCIENCE™

Selection of our books indexed in the Book Citation Index in Web of Science™ Core Collection (BKCI)

Interested in publishing with us?
Contact book.department@intechopen.com

Numbers displayed above are based on latest data collected.
For more information visit www.intechopen.com

For EU product safety concerns:
IN TECH d.o.o., Prolaz Marije Krucifikse Kozulić 3, 51000 Rijeka, Croatia,
info@intechopen.com or visit our website at intechopen.com.

Meet the editor

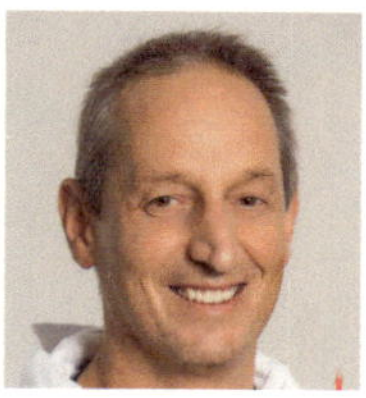

Prof. Endre Zima, MD, Ph.D., is the chief of the cardiac ICU at Semmelweis University Heart and Vascular Center, Budapest, Hungary. He is a consultant in anesthesiology, intensive care, and cardiology. He achieved a Ph.D. and a medical habilitation degree from Semmelweis University in 2006 and 2017, respectively. As a professor, he holds graduate and postgraduate lectures and practices in anesthesiology, intensive care and cardiology. He is a full Instructor of the European Resuscitation Council in Advanced Life Support (ALS) and Basic Life Support (BLS). Dr. Zima is a fellow of the European Society of Cardiology, the European Heart Rhythm Association (EHRA), and the Acute Cardiovascular Care Association. He achieved the EHRA accreditation for Cardiac Pacing and Implantable Cardioverter Defibrillators. He is past president of the Working Group on Cardiac Arrhythmias and Pacing and board member of the Hungarian Society of Cardiology and Working Group of Heart Failure. He is a member of the Hungarian Society of Resuscitation and the Hungarian Society of Anesthesiology and Intensive Therapy. He has developed protocols for cardiac intensive care and anesthesia for special critical cardiac procedures, such as treatment of cardiogenic shock, electrical storm, protocol of target temperature management (TTM) of post-cardiac arrest syndrome (PCAS), anesthesia for ablations, transcatheter aortic valve replacement (TAVR), subcutaneous implantable cardioverter defibrillator (S-ICD), barostimulator implantations, and more. His fields of research are cardiopulmonary resuscitation, post-cardiac arrest intensive care, arrhythmias, ICDs/implantable pulse generators (IPGs), cardiac resynchronization therapy (CRT) therapy, defibrillator development, acute and intensive cardiac care, cardiogenic shock/acute heart failure, and invasive hemodynamic monitoring. He is currently supervising the scientific research work of four Ph.D. students and three medical students. Professor Zima and his co-authors have two accepted patents to their credit. He is the author of thirteen book chapters, sixty-six international journal articles, and fifty-six native-language papers (26 papers in D1, and 46 in Q1 category) with a total citation of 3234, Hirsch-index of 18, g-index of 27.

Contents

Preface

Updates on Cardiac Defibrillation, Cardioversion and AED Development delves deeply into the world of cardiac tachyarrhythmia treatment. Through various approaches, the chapters detail special arrays of electrical and pharmacological methods to prevent tachyarrhythmias or to convert tachyarrhythmia to normal rhythm.

Chapter 1, "Cardioversion" by Mevlut Demir, discusses the procedure of cardioversion, which employs electrical or medical methods to restore normal sinus rhythm during tachyarrhythmic events. Electrical cardioversion, employing QRS-synchronized direct current is the favored approach for tachyarrhythmias with QRS complexes when pharmacological interventions fail or hemodynamic instability occurs. The chapter also highlights its differentiation from defibrillation, focusing on common indications such as atrial fibrillation and flutter while cautioning against its use in certain cases.

Chapter 2, "History of the Development of Automated External Defibrillators", by Oskars Kalejs et al., raises curiosity about the historical journey that led to these life-saving devices becoming commonplace. The chapter's structure as a historical excursion invites readers to explore the evolution of cardiac electrical therapies, particularly defibrillation. It also depicts the pioneers behind it and the progression of AEDs from initial concepts to their pivotal role in modern resuscitation.

Chapter 3, "ICD for Sudden Cardiac Death Prevention and New Pharmaceutical Treatment Options in Hypertrophic Obstructive Cardiomyopathy", by Antonio da Silva Menezes Junior et al., discusses the intricate nature of hypertrophic cardiomyopathy (HCM), primarily caused by autosomal dominant sarcomeric gene mutations, resulting in reduced heart compliance, myofibrillar disarray, and fibrosis. The chapter highlights evolved management strategies that enable HCM patients to expect a normal lifespan without invasive interventions. While curative treatments for hypertrophy and heart dysfunction are lacking, drug-based therapies aim to alleviate symptoms and decelerate disease progression. The study introduces mavacamten, a reversible cardiac myosin allosteric modulator showing promising potential for improving obstructive HCM patients' health. Crucially, implantable cardioverter-defibrillators are pivotal for preventing sudden cardiac death in HCM cases, alongside the challenges of managing atrial arrhythmias and the growing utilization of anti-arrhythmic drugs and, as least resort, radiofrequency ablations.

Chapter 4, "Atrial Fibrillation and Cardioversion Drugs", by Taomin Su et al., addresses the detrimental impact of atrial arrhythmias, particularly tachyarrhythmias, on heart function and their potential contribution to heart failure. Atrial fibrillation, a prominent type of atrial arrhythmia, is characterized by disrupted atrial contractions and is a prevalent and serious condition in clinical practice, associated with significant complications such as hemodynamic alterations and systemic thromboembolism. Consequently, the study emphasizes the significance of developing new and more effective cardioversion drugs as a key focus in arrhythmia research.

Chapter 5, "AED: Optimal Use of Automated External Defribilators in BLS and ILS", by Tudor Ovidiu Popa et al., addresses the challenge of effectively managing cardiac arrests, particularly in adults, through the use of Automated External Defibrillators (AEDs) in public-access defibrillation programs during cardiopulmonary resuscitation (CPR). While the majority of adult out-of-hospital cardiac arrests result from ventricular fibrillation, training laypersons in Basic Life Support (BLS) and AED usage can significantly increase survival rates. Despite the rise in public-access AEDs, the low ratio of lay-rescuer AED utilization and bystander CPR proficiency underscores the need for continuous training and public awareness to optimize outcomes in cardiac arrest scenarios.

Chapter 6, "The Influence of Transthoracic Impedance on Electrical Cardioversion and Defibrillation: Current Data", by Ádam Pál-Jakab et al., focuses on the prevailing emergency treatment in clinical practice such as electrical cardioversion (ECV) and direct current defibrillation (DF) that offer rapid, effective, and safe treatments for hemodynamically unstable cardiac arrhythmias. By definition, the success of both ECV and DF depends on the delivered shock energy that is determined by current output and transthoracic impedance (TTI). While factors such as respiration, contact pressure, and energy delivered influence ECV and DF success, conflicting results of studies regarding predictors of TTI, such as age and gender, persist. The chapter reviews the potential strategies for optimizing ECV and DF efficacy by adjusting the delivered energy based on individual variables affecting thoracic impedance, offering the potential for prediction system-driven automated energy optimization.

Endre Zima
Department of Cardiology,
Semmelweis University Heart and Vascular Centre,
Budapest, Hungary

Section 1

Cardioversion and Defibrillation

Chapter 1

Cardioversion

Mevlut Demir

Abstract

Cardioversion (CV) is a procedure consisting of 2 different applications, electrical or medical, performed to provide normal sinus rhythm in arrhythmic events. Electrical cardioversion is the preferred direct current-mediated treatment for arrhythmia without sinus rhythm when there is no response to pharmacological therapy or hemodynamic instability due to tachycardia. The difference between defibrillation and electrical cardioversion; in electrical cardioversion, direct current is given on the R or S wave in the QRS by synchronizing with electrocardiography, and in defibrillation, it is given at any moment of the cardiac cycle. Atrial fibrillation and flutter are the most common arrhythmias in which cardioversion is used. Electrical cardioversion should not be performed in patients with ventricular fibrillation, pulseless ventricular tachycardia and digital poisoning. After cardioversion, temporary ST segment elevations, thromboembolism, ventricular fibrillation, short-term bradycardia/asystole, hypotension, pulmonary edema and elevation of cardiac enzymes that do not constitute clinical significance can be observed.

Keywords: atrial fibrillation, atrial flutter, cardioversion, electrotherapy, supraventricular tachycardia, synchronized, ventricular tachycardia

1. Introduction

Cardioversion (CV) is a procedure consisting of 2 different applications, electrical or medical, performed to provide normal sinus rhythm in arrhythmic events. While medical cardioversion is preferred in stable patients and often in elective patients, electrical cardioversion is often preferred in patients who cannot get a medical response or who need an urgent CV [1, 2].

Electrical cardioversion has played an important role for the last 6 decades in the treatment of arrhythmias via direct current today. About 15 years after defibrillation, which was first performed in humans in 1947, electrical cardioversion was applied to convert AF and VT to normal sinus rhythm. Synchronized cardioversion is a procedure similar to defibrillation performed to terminate a life-threatening or hemodynamically unstable tachycardic arrhythmia. The difference between defibrillation and electrical cardioversion; in electrical cardioversion, direct current is given on the R or S wave in the QRS by synchronizing with the electrocardiography, and in defibrillation, it is given at any time of the cardiac cycle. The purpose of synchronization; the aim is to avoid the delivery of energy on the T wave, which coincides with the sensitive period of the myocardium, which may trigger VF. The appropriate approach in cardioversion is to start cardioversion with the recommended energy levels in specific arrhythmias (e.g. initial shock for atrial flutter 70–120 joule) [3–6].

2. Indications

As a general rule, synchronous cardioversion is the preferred treatment for tachycardia without sinus rhythm, when there is no response to pharmacological treatment, or when hemodynamics due to tachycardia worsens. In contrast to the defibrillation used in cardiac arrest patients, emergency synchronized cardioversion is performed in patients who still have a pulse but are hemodynamically unstable. It is also used to treat hemodynamically unstable ventricular and supraventricular rhythms [3, 4].

The following are the most common indications;

- Atrial fibrillation- flutter
- Supraventricular tachycardia due to reentry
- Atrial tachycardia
- Ventricular tachycardia with pulse

Atrial fibrillation and flutter are the most common arrhythmias in which cardioversion is used. Whether rhythm control or rate control should be provided in AF patients is still a controversial issue. However, if the patient is stable and a rhythm control decision has been made, first of all, heart rate control should be provided, and then cardioversion should be planned by making appropriate preparations after anticoagulation at the effective dose and time.

In patients with AF whose duration is unknown or lasts longer than 48 hours, left atrial/appendix thrombus should be ruled out by transesophageal echocardiography before, otherwise effective anticoagulation should be performed for at least 3 weeks before the procedure, and cardioversion should be planned afterwards. Because of the time interval required for recovery of atrial mechanical functions after cardioversion, anticoagulation should be continued for at least 4 weeks even if sinus rhythm is achieved. In patients who are sure to have AF of less than 48 hours, cardioversion can be performed by applying anticoagulation before the procedure. Anticoagulants should be continued for at least 4 weeks [5, 7–10].

It has been shown that biphasic devices and anteroposterior electrode positions for atrial fibrillation cardioversion are more effective with lower energy, and the recommended energy is 120–200 joules for biphasic waveforms. If it fails, the process can be repeated by increasing to higher energies. In AF patients, long duration of AF (especially longer than 1 year), increased left atrial dimensions, mitral valve disease, obesity, and chronic obstructive pulmonary disease are factors that decrease the success rate of cardioversion or increase the likelihood of recurrence. Premedication before cardioversion (with amiodarone- ibutilide), the use of a biphasic device and anteroposterior application are approaches that increase the chances of success of cardioversion [5, 8, 10].

In atrial flutter, the anticoagulant approach is the same as AF and it is recommended to start with lower energy levels, biphasic 70–120 joules, monophasic 100 joules due to a more organized arrhythmia [3, 11, 12].

Supraventricular tachyarrhythmias are often terminated with vagal maneuvers or with a medical approach. But if there is no response to them or in case of hemodynamic instability, cardioversion can be performed with a high success rate by starting with 50–100 joules. Routine anticoagulation before cardioversion is not required in SVT patients [3, 13].

In patients with stable hemodynamics, besides ventricular tachycardia with pulse, an approach with medical antiarrhythmic therapy can be planned first under close follow-up. However, emergency cardioversion should be performed in cases of hemodynamic instability, signs of heart failure, angina, and changes in mental status. Organized arrhythmias, such as monomorphic VT, are easily picked up with lower energy levels, while non-organized multiple focal arrhythmias such as polymorphic VT or VF and large myocardial arrhythmias require higher energy levels. In monomorphic VT, it is recommended to start with 100 joules with a biphasic device and 200 joules with a monophasic device, while in polymorphic VT, it is recommended to start with 150–200 joules with a biphasic device and 200–360 joules with a monophasic device. Routine anticoagulation before cardioversion is also not required in VT patients [3–5, 7].

3. Contraindications

Cardioversion should not be performed in patients with ventricular fibrillation and pulseless VT, defibrillation should definitely be performed [3].

Increased automaticity or triggered activity-induced arrhythmias, junctional tachycardia (e.g. digoxin intoxication), accelerated idioventricular rhythm, multifocal atrial tachycardia, and sinus tachycardia in cardioversion are not indicated. Even tachyarrhythmias due to endogenous catecholamine release may be aggravated after cardioversion. In digital poisoning, the excitability of the myocardium increases, and cardioversion is contraindicated, as it can cause resistant VF. However, it is not necessary to discontinue the drug before cardioversion in patients using digital who do not have clinical signs of digital toxicity. Cardioversion should also not be performed in stable AF patients who have not taken optimal anticoagulants or whose left atrial thrombus has not been ruled out with TEE [3, 5, 7, 9, 14].

4. Procedure

Preparation before cardioversion in stable patients will both increase the chances of success of the procedure, make the patient less traumatized, and reduce the likelihood of complications for the physician. Serum electrolytes should be checked before starting the procedure, and secondary causes that may exacerbate tachycardia (hyperthyroidism, anemia, etc.) should be reviewed. The recommended steps for successful cardioversion are described below (**Figure 1**).

- Except for unstable patients, the patient should be informed and approval should be obtained before the procedure.

- Patients should be fasted about 6–8 hours before the elective procedure.

- Resuscitation equipment must be available at the patient's bedside.

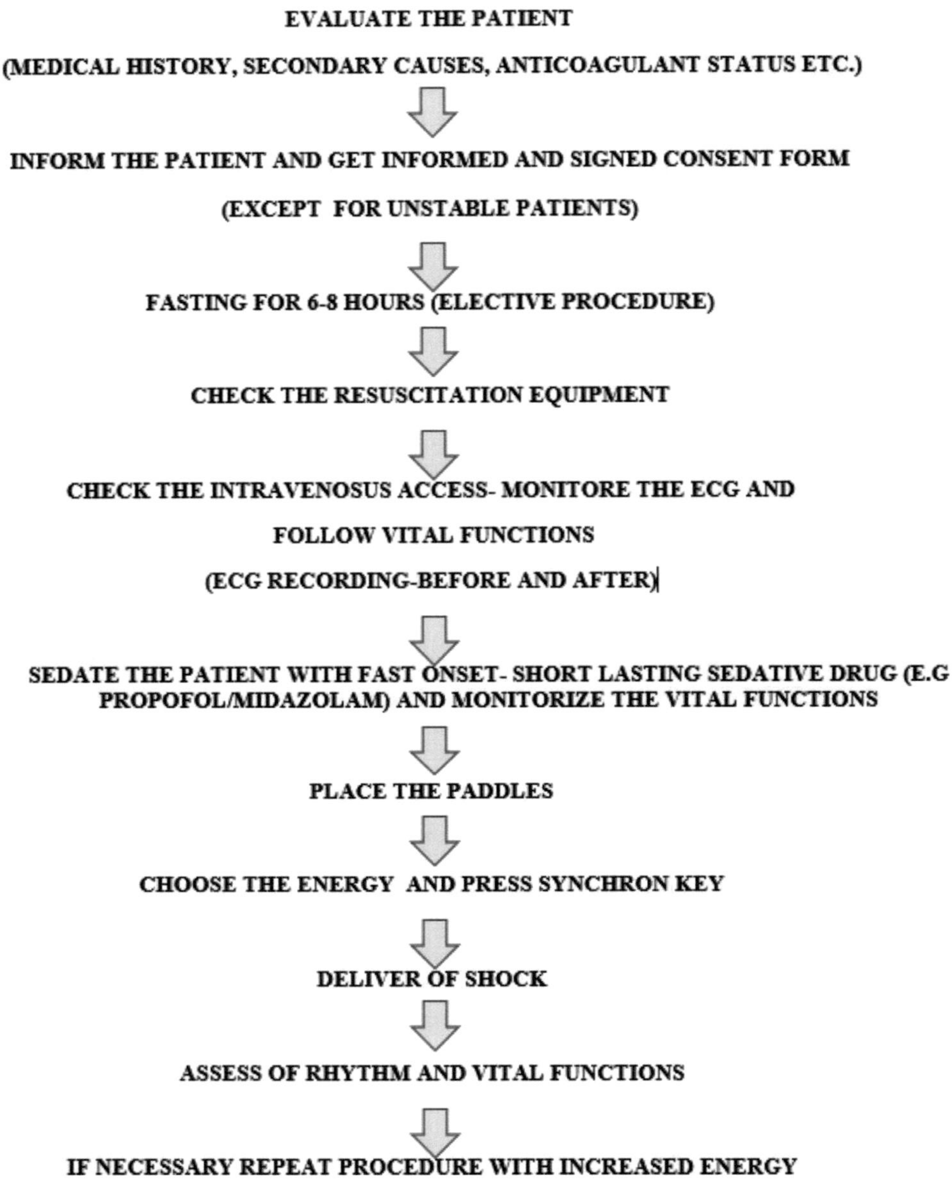

Figure 1.
Practical algorithm for cardioversion.

- The airway patency of the patients, continuous ECG monitoring, and active vascular access should be absolutely checked.
- A 12-lead ECG should be seen before and after the procedure.
- Sedation with fast-onset-short-lasting drugs (such as midazolam, propofol) is recommended before elective cardioversion.
- Selection of the biphasic device, optimal use of the gel, and placement of the paddles by pressing and discharge in expiration are the factors that can increase the chance of success.

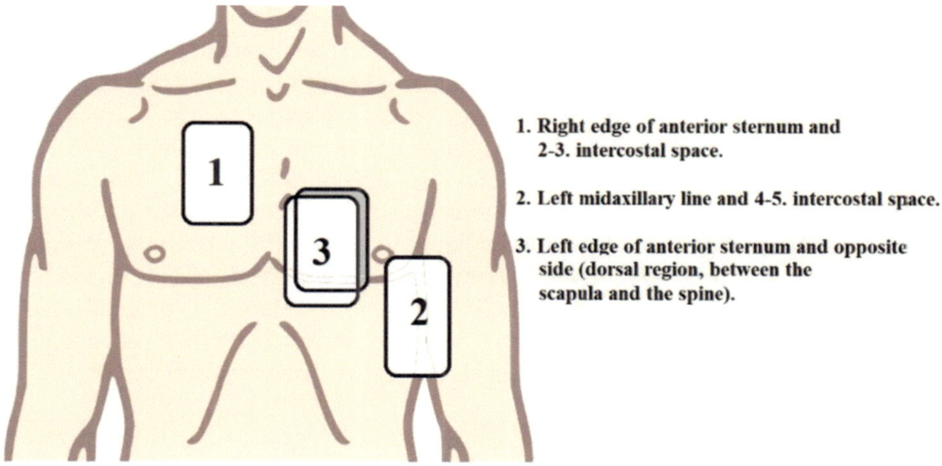

Figure 2.
Localization of paddles.

- The paddles should be placed in the appropriate localization (**Figure 2**. Localization 1–2 for anterolateral (apex-anterior), 3 and opposite side for anteroposterior), and the SYNCHRON key must be pressed before the procedure. If there is no response in the first shock, the process should be continued by increasing the energy level.

5. Complications

After cardioversion, arrhythmias that do not require treatment, short-term bradycardia/asystole (especially in antiarrhythmic users, the elderly, long-term AF patients), and ST-T changes may be observed frequently. Bradyarrhythmia that requires temporary pacemakers may develop, especially in patients with acute coronary syndrome. ST elevation lasting under 2 minutes can be monitored. Rarely, VF can also be triggered by proper cardioversion. It has been reported that embolic cerebrovascular accident develops in 1–3% of AF patients after sinus rhythm is achieved. If a healthcare worker comes into contact during the application, the healthcare worker may be affected. In addition, especially due to inappropriate technique, skin burns may be seen in the areas that come into contact directly after the current, creams for the burn can be used. Side effects, hypotension, and hypoventilation may be observed due to the sedation agent applied before the procedure. Rarely, hypotension, pulmonary edema, and elevation of cardiac enzymes that do not constitute clinical significance can be observed [1, 5, 7, 9, 15].

6. Special cases

Supraventricular tachycardia and atrial fibrillation are the most common arrhythmias in pregnancy. Electrical CV is also used as the first choice for maneuvering medically unresponsive and unstable patients. When the literature is reviewed, it can be said that cardioversion is safe for both mother and fetus during pregnancy and is the same approach as in normal adults [7, 16].

It has been reported that the frequency of complications due to electrical cardioversion performed in patients with pacemakers or ICD develops rarely. In patients who developed complications, temporary pacing or sensitivity threshold changes were often observed. In order to detect and avoid these complications, it is recommended to check the battery and lead first. Then it is recommended to program the battery's voltage output to a higher, program it to VOO or AOO mode. The pedals should be placed 15 cm away from the generator and the direction of the paddles should be placed in the position perpendicular to the endocardial leads. A 5-minute time interval should be given between the two shock waves. Lead and pacemaker control should be performed again after CV. The threshold should be programmed as higher for at least 4–6 weeks, and then the battery and lead should be checked again. In case of a suspected problem, earlier control and intervention can be planned [5, 7, 17, 18].

7. Conclusion

Cardioversion is still a treatment method that has an important place in the treatment of arrhythmias and can be applied in emergency or elective patients. In cardioversion, from the patient selection to the appropriate energy use, from the use of gel to anticoagulant therapy, many of the above-mentioned factors affect the success and complications of cardioversion. Therefore, although it may seem simple, it is a procedure that every stage of it should be carefully followed for high success and low complication.

Author details

Mevlut Demir
Department of Cardiology, Kutahya Health Science University, Kutahya, Turkey

*Address all correspondence to: mevlut.demir@ksbu.edu.tr

IntechOpen

© 2023 The Author(s). Licensee IntechOpen. This chapter is distributed under the terms of the Creative Commons Attribution License (http://creativecommons.org/licenses/by/3.0), which permits unrestricted use, distribution, and reproduction in any medium, provided the original work is properly cited.

References

[1] Jordan JR, Manogue M, Williams BR III. Cardioversion. In: McKean SC, Ross JJ, Dressler DD, Scheurer DB, editors. Principles and Practice of Hospital Medicine, 2e [Internet]. New York, NY: McGraw-Hill Education; 2017. Available from: http://www.accessmedicine.mhmedical.com/content.aspx?aid=1137614050

[2] Valentinuzzi ME, Arriascu LS. Electrical cardioversion: A review. International Journal of Clinical Cardiology. 2020;**7**:164

[3] Link MS, Atkins DL, Passman RS, Halperin HR, Samson RA, White RD, et al. Part 6: Electrical therapies: Automated external defibrillators, defibrillation, cardioversion, and pacing: 2010 American Heart Association guidelines for cardiopulmonary resuscitation and emergency cardiovascular care. Circulation. 2010;**122**(18 Suppl. 3):S706-S719

[4] Lown B. Defibrillation and Cardioversion. Cardiovascular Research. Vol. 55. no. 2. Amsterdam: Elservier Science; 2002. pp. 220-224

[5] Miller JM, Tomaselli GF, Zipes DP. Therapy for cardiac arrhythmias. Braunwald's heart disease: A textbook of cardiovascular medicine 10th edition Saunders. BMH Medical Journal-ISSN 2348-392X. 2018;**5**(2):670-705

[6] Lown B, Amarasingham R, Neuman J. New method for terminating cardiac arrhythmias. Use of synchronized capacitor discharge. JAMA. 1962;**182**:548-555

[7] Sucu M, Davutoglu V, Ozer O. Electrical cardioversion. Annals of Saudi Medicine. 2009;**29**(3):201-206

[8] Fornengo C, Antolini M, Frea S, Gallo C, Grosso Marra W, Morello M, et al. Prediction of atrial fibrillation recurrence after cardioversion in patients with left-atrial dilation. European Heart Journal-Cardiovascular Imaging. 2015;**16**(3):335-341

[9] Nusair M, Flaker GC, Chockalingam A. Electric cardioversion of atrial fibrillation. Missouri Medicine. 2010;**107**(1):59

[10] Hindrics G, Potpara T, Dagres N. ESC guidelines for the diagnosis and management of atrial fibrillation with the Eukropean Association for Cardio-Thoracic Surgery (EACTS): The task force for the diagonosis and management of atrial fibrillation of the ESC developer with the secial contribution of the European heart Rythm association (EHRA) of the ESC. European Heart Journal. 2021;**42**:373-498

[11] Saliba W, Juratli N, Chung MK, Niebauer MJ, Erdogan O, Trohman R, et al. Higher energy synchronized external direct current cardioversion for refractory atrial fibrillation. Journal of the American College of Cardiology. 1999;**34**(7):2031-2034

[12] Soar J, Böttiger BW, Carli P, Couper K, Deakin CD, Djärv T, et al. European resuscitation council guidelines 2021: Adult advanced life support. Resuscitation. 2021;**161**:115-151

[13] Katritsis DG, Arbelo E, Arribas F, Bax JJ, Blomstrom-Lundqvist C, Calkins H, et al. 2019 ESC guidelines for the management of patients with supraventricular tachycardia. European Heart Journal. 2020;**41**:655À720

[14] Bertaglia E, Anselmino M, Zorzi A, Russo V, Toso E, Peruzza F, et al. NOACs and atrial fibrillation: Incidence and predictors of left atrial thrombus in the real world. International Journal of Cardiology. 2017;**249**:179-183

[15] Cemin R, Rauhe W, Marini M, Pescoller F, Pitscheider W. Serum troponin I level after external electrical direct current synchronized cardioversion in patients with normal or reduced ejection fraction: no evidence of myocytes injury. Clinical Cardiology: An International Indexed and Peer-Reviewed Journal for Advances in the Treatment of Cardiovascular Disease. 2005;**28**(10):467-470

[16] Pacheco JAH, Angel NTM, Rojo LB, Marenco MEL. Electrical and pharmacological cardioversion during pregnancy: Case series and literature review. Annals of Clinical Case Reports. 2021;**6**:2025

[17] Lüker J, Sultan A, Plenge T, van den Bruck J, Heeger CH, Meyer S, et al. Electrical cardioversion of patients with implanted pacemaker or cardioverter–defibrillator: Results of a survey of german centers and systematic review of the literature. Clinical Research in Cardiology. 2018;**107**:249-258

[18] Waller C, Callies F, Langenfeld H. Adverse effects of direct current cardioversion on cardiac pacemakers and electrodes: Is external cardioversion contraindicated in patients with permanent pacing systems? EP Europace. 2004;**6**(2):165-168

Chapter 2

History of the Development of Automated External Defibrillators

Oskars Kalejs, Aija Maca-Kaleja, Ketija Apsite, Anita Abula and Laura Strazdina

Abstract

This chapter is structured as a historical overview of the history of the development of defibrillators and the most prominent personalities who contributed to the development of the modern concept of resuscitation. Defibrillators in medical practice can be external or implanted. The devices, known as automated external defibrillators, automate the diagnosis of a patient's rhythm and the process of stopping arrhythmias, meaning they can be used successfully by nonspecialists. In Europe, 350,000–700,000 people suffer from sudden cardiac arrest every year. On average, it is 55–113 per 100,000 people. Most of these people are usually at home, but about 10–20% of victims are in a public place at the time. Defibrillation within 3–5 minutes of cardiac arrest can increase survival by 50–70%. For every minute that defibrillation is delayed, the chance of survival decreases by 10–12%. A significant contribution to the development of the defibrillation concept was made by Peter Kristians Abildgård, Albert Salisbury Hyman, William Bennett Couwenhoven, Paul Morris Zoll, James Francis Pantridge, and many others. Clinical studies confirm that public access defibrillators (PADs), when available and used correctly during out-of-hospital cardiac arrest, were associated with a 40% median survival rate.

Keywords: history of defibrillators, sudden cardiac death, resuscitation, automated external defibrillators, public access defibrillation

1. Introduction

To us, people living in the twenty-first century, many things seem self-evident. Both various household electronics, transcontinental flights, space exploration, and much more. We take medical advances, including rapid advances in resuscitation options and automated external defibrillators available in public places, as a matter of course. Whether it is an airport or a railway station, a gym or a large store, the existence of such a device and its easy identification seems completely normal. You see the classic sign of an Automated external defibrillator (AED), and it triggers no emotions – this is the norm as it should be. However, at such moments, interest arises – how long did science need to develop, so that these great devices, which have saved thousands of lives, have become a self-explanatory part of your everyday life? Who are the people who took the first steps in their invention, research and did so much to

IntechOpen

make the concepts of "defibrillation," "cardioversion," "resuscitation" not something unknown and exotic anymore but completely normal? Historical aspects have always been fascinating, both in architecture, linguistics, and culture. The same can be said about medical science. Medical development has been focused on preserving human life and health for many thousands of years. Unfortunately, clinical medicine often encounters acute and urgent situations where every second counts, and a person's life depends on quick and professional action. What has this path been like? What personalities have contributed to AED being a classic every day? About that and a few other things in this chapter.

The authors chose to structure this chapter as a historical excursion, in which we invite you to walk with us through the history of defibrillation and the creation of defibrillators, to dwell on the personalities, and to look at the first clinical studies and further development of AED.

2. The concepts of "defibrillation" and "synchronized cardioversion"

What do we mean by the terms "defibrillation" and "synchronized cardioversion"? What is the basis of the defibrillation process? What changes are caused by defibrillation? About it in this subsection.

2.1 Defibrillation

Defibrillation is a treatment for life-threatening heart rhythm disorders, especially ventricular fibrillation (VF) and ventricular tachycardia (VT). A defibrillator delivers a dose of electrical current (often called a defibrillator) to the heart. Although not fully understood, this process depolarizes the heart muscle cells, stopping an existing arrhythmia. After the depolarization, the body's natural pacemaker – the rhythm generation cells of the conduction system in the heart's sinoatrial node are able to restore normal sinus rhythm. A heart in asystole (isoelectric line on the ECG) cannot be restarted with a defibrillator but can only be treated with cardiopulmonary resuscitation (CPR) and intravenous vasopressors such as epinephrine (adrenaline).

Defibrillators in medical practice can be external, transvenous, or implanted (implantable cardioverter-defibrillator), depending on the type of device used or required. Some external devices, known as automated external defibrillators (AEDs), automate the diagnosis of the patient's rhythms, which means that they can be used successfully by nonspecialists either after a short training course (security personnel, sports complex instructors, flight crews, police officers, etc.) or without that provided by the algorithms built into these machines for fully automatic operation.

2.2 Synchronized electrical cardioversion

Unlike defibrillation, synchronized electrical cardioversion is an electrical shock that is delivered by synchronizing the shock with the heart's cycle. Although the person may still be in a critical condition, the goal of cardioversion is usually to stop cardiac arrhythmias that result in significant impairment of circulation and perfusion, such as ventricular tachycardia or atrial flutter, or atrial fibrillation.

The defibrillator system generates a rapid discharge of electric current, depolarizing most of the heart muscle quickly (practically instantly). One could even say that the simultaneous depolarization puts the action potential in the 0 state in most myocardial cells. The effect of this energy discharge, which is often referred to as a "shock," interrupts the electrical activity of chaotic cells, and stops the inefficient operation of the heart. The term used to describe this inefficient and chaotic cellular activity is "fibrillation," successively stopping this process is called "defibrillation." After complete depolarization, there is a period in which the electrical activity of the heart is at zero level, but after this pause, cells of the sinus node start to work as the highest centers of rhythm generation of the cardiac conduction system, or in some cases, the cells of the rhythm generation system of the secondary level or substitute levels are activated. Consequently, the normal physiological sequence and synchronicity of the heart rhythm is restored.

After defibrillation is performed, in the optimal version, it returns to normal sinus rhythm, where it begins to provide physiological circulation in the body, ensuring that oxygen-rich blood reaches cells throughout the body. Skin color may return to normal, oxygenation improves, and in some cases, the person will also spontaneously recover other life-sustaining functions as physiological circulation is restored.

Defibrillation stops the heart's electrical activity and allows the action potential of its pacemaker cells to fire. The effectiveness of the procedure depends on the metabolic state of the myocardium (due to the cause and time of heart failure) and the correct realization of the defibrillation protocol.

2.3 What is the defibrillation mechanism?

Extracellular electric current shocks are widely used to treat ventricular tachyarrhythmias. Extracellular current flow induced by defibrillation shocks is thought to produce changes in membrane potential (ΔVm); these changes then interrupt reentrant circuits, prolonging ventricular refractoriness, and/or generating new waves of excitation. The defibrillation shock causes depolarization or hyperpolarization, which takes place in the ventricular myocardium and which is located at a relatively large distance from the surface electrodes used in the defibrillation process. Several mechanisms are known that most likely explain such limited ΔVm formation. When performing myocardial mapping with the application of continuous linear leads, the parameters of ΔVm are limited to the area located in the immediate vicinity of the discharge electrodes. Such a region, whose dimensions exceed ≈3 length constants, is defined as the "close-field" or "polarity region." The resulting ΔVm, labeled "primary source." When analyzing secondary sources, i.e., those located within ΔVm (>2 to 3 mm) of the electrical discharge electrodes, such a situation may arise if the current flowing during the shock is forced to divide locally between the extracellular and intracellular environments. Such a distribution can be caused by a number of factors such as systemic electrical changes in electrical connections between myocardial cells, changes in cell order or myocardial fiber geometry, heterogeneity of the extracellular space and associated resistance changes, as well as anisotropy-induced changes in the resistance ratio of intracellular and extracellular systems, also denoted as "bidomain effect."

2.4 Why is this topic so relevant?

In Europe, 350,000–700,000 persons suffer sudden cardiac arrest every year. On average, it is 55–113 per 100,000 people. In Latvia, on average, around 1500 people have a sudden cardiac arrest during the year. Most of these people are usually at home, but it also happens in public places – about 10–20% of the victims are currently in a public place – an airport, a supermarket, a public institution, or a sports center.

When you are with a person who has suffered a sudden cardiac arrest, it is important to make a decision in the first few seconds and provide help in the first few minutes. Although the first aid provider himself does not realize it at all, the health and even life of the patient depends on his correct actions.

The most important thing in sudden cardiac arrest is to provide continuous chest compressions. Chest compressions achieve continuous blood supply to the entire body. However, chest compressions are not always enough.

About 20–50% of all sudden cardiac arrests are those that can be treated with electrophysiological therapy, or defibrillation. The importance of defibrillation has been particularly emphasized in recent years – it has been scientifically proven that every minute in which defibrillation is not performed decreases the patient's survival by 7–10%.

3. Briefly about AED

3.1 Automated external defibrillator (AED)

AEDs are portable devices that automatically analyze the heart rhythm of patients in cardiac arrest and deliver a shock, or defibrillation, if ventricular fibrillation or ventricular tachycardia is detected. Rhythm diagnosis is not part of the competence of peer assistance. The only difference between a shockable and a nonshockable rhythm is the AED's audible message, which will say "shock advised," indicating that the device has detected either VF or VT.

As previously mentioned, defibrillation within 3–5 minutes of loss of consciousness can increase survival by 50–70%. For every minute that defibrillation is delayed, the probability of survival decreases by 10–12%. Early defibrillation can be achieved by first responder use of publicly available automated external defibrillators. This type of approach should be implemented in public places with high population density, such as airports, railway stations, bus stations, sports arenas, shopping malls, or in places where there has been one case of cardiac arrest in 5 years. A record of previous such events (cardiac arrests) in a given area, as well as neighborhood characteristics, can help determine the most appropriate AED placement.

Both audio instructions and graphic instructions on the device are used to operate and operate the AED. The devices are safe and effective and designed for use by both trained and untrained people. AEDs allow rapid defibrillation for several minutes before receiving professional help. The helper should focus on following the voice instructions and continue to act according to the instructions. Standard AEDs are suitable for use on victims who have reached the age of 8 years.

AED designs may vary by manufacturer, but the basic components are the same for these devices. The user is instructed to turn on the device and expose the victim's chest. The paddles of the device must be opened and removed from the protective base, then placed on the victim's chest according to the AED graphic so that the heart rhythm can be detected and a discharge can be performed if necessary. Background motion can affect the accuracy of the result, so providers are instructed to stop CPR during rhythm analysis. International standards require AED sensitivity to detect VF >90% (VF at least 0.2 mV amplitude) and overall specificity >95%.

Most AEDs deliver 120–350 J of power. The choice of power depends on several factors, including the number of previous defibrillations and the resistance of the chest wall. AEDs typically provide audio instructions that prompt responders to stand away from the victim during rhythm analysis and press a button to deliver the shock. The AED is programmed to perform a rhythm analysis every 2 minutes and also instructs the rescuer to continue CPR.

Another important aspect that can affect survival in cardiac arrest is the registration of AEDs for public access and the availability of information to call dispatchers so that responders can be directed to the nearest AED {Ringh, 2018, The challenges and possibilities of public access defibrillation} if necessary [1].

ILCOR has developed an AED identification mark/marking that is recognized worldwide (see **Figure 1**).

ILCOR (*The International Liaison Committee on Resuscitation*) is an international cooperation committee whose goal is to promote the creation of common protocols for collaborative resuscitation and emergency medical care. The internationally accepted abbreviations CPR (Cardiopulmonary Resuscitation) and ECC (Emergency Cardiovascular Care) are used to denote the protocols. The organization was established in 1992. ILCOR includes professional associations and organizations such as the American Heart Association (AHA), the European Resuscitation Council (ERC), the Heart and Stroke Foundation of Canada (HSFC), the Australian and New Zealand Committee on Resuscitation (ANZCOR), the Resuscitation Council of South Africa (RCSA), the Asian Resuscitation Council (RCA), Inter American Heart Foundation (IAHF). Interestingly, the name of the organization is formed from the compound "ill cor," which means a sick heart; in Latin "cor" means heart.

A significant practical obstacle to using an AED is that, in this case, at least two helpers are needed – one to perform CPR and the other to obtain the AED.

One of the strategies for more effective attraction of fellow citizens provides that, while the emergency medical service (EMS) is being called, the instructions for

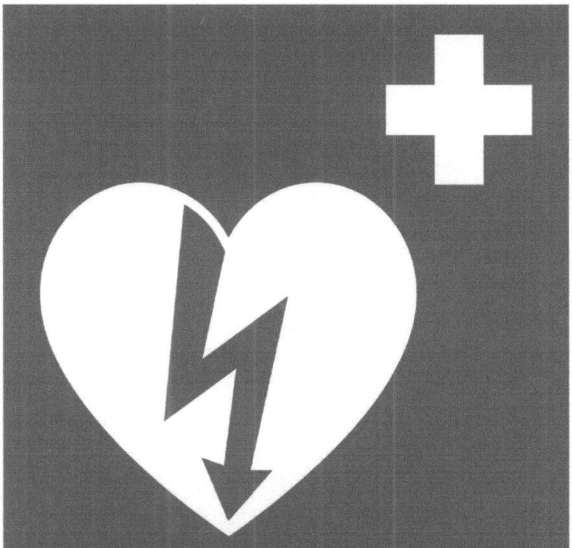

Figure 1.
International AED designation [2].

providing help are additionally given over the phone, and during this time, the dispatchers can warn other members of the public about such a case with the help of messaging or a special phone application. This approach allows for the notification of people who have volunteered for such digital transmission of information in the event of a cardiac arrest, thereby obtaining information about the event, its location, and, in some cases, the nearest publicly available AED. Although this is a new strategy, early studies have shown an increase in the rate of early initiation of CPR and the associated survival rate. Such a strategy is officially supported by the AHA.

Finally, a dispatcher may be able to send an AED to the scene by drone. This approach is still being researched, but early modeling of the system indicates that an AED can be delivered to the scene significantly faster by drone than by standard EMS transport, reducing time to the scene by 6 minutes in urban settings and 19 minutes outside of urban settings.

The potential lifesaving benefits of AEDs in public settings have been extensively studied. A review of several studies of public access defibrillation noted that the average number of patients who survived hospital discharge was 53% when defibrillated by bystanders compared with 28.6% of patients who survived when defibrillated by EMS personnel.

A 2018 study compared bystander defibrillation with an AED and defibrillation by an EMS specialist. The study examined nearly 50,000 cardiac arrests in 9 United States regions. According to the study, 66.5% of patients who were defibrillated by a bystander, compared to 43% of patients who were defibrillated by EMS personnel, survived to hospital discharge. In addition, it was found that at the time of discharge, a better neurological outcome was more often observed in patients who were defibrillated by peers (57.1 and 32.7%, respectively). Among all reported out-of-hospital cardiac arrests, an AED was used in 15.9% of cases. The benefit of bystander defibrillation with an AED increased with increasing time to EMS arrival [3].

Although AEDs offer many advantages and are essential in providing assistance, there are several challenges to their availability. For example, many AEDs are located in public places such as schools, business offices, and sports centers that are not accessible to the public at night or on weekends. One example is Toronto, where the total number of registered AEDs is 737, of which 707 were available during the middle of the day, and 228 or 30.9% were available at night [4].

3.2 Why is this topic so relevant?

Sudden cardiac arrest is one of the leading causes of death in Europe and worldwide. For a large number of people, cardiac arrest occurs outside the hospital, when first aid can be provided by fellow citizens. The number of people who survive OHCA (Out-of-Hospital Cardiac Arrest) varies around 10% in Europe [2]. The most important thing is the ability to recognize this condition and to initiate a set of assistance in time. In order to improve the survival abilities of these people, fellow citizens must act immediately – it is necessary to call emergency medical help and start cardiopulmonary resuscitation measures, which include chest compressions and breathing.

In recent years, the topic of the use of AEDs in such cases has been brought up, and various studies have been conducted to clarify their effectiveness and the involvement of fellow human beings in the use of these devices. An AED is a device that performs a defibrillation function and can be used by nonmedical personnel. It has been shown that early defibrillation in cases of cardiac arrest, when it is needed, reduces the victim's probability of survival until discharge from the hospital by 10–12%.

DOI: http://dx.doi.org/10.5772/intechopen.112518

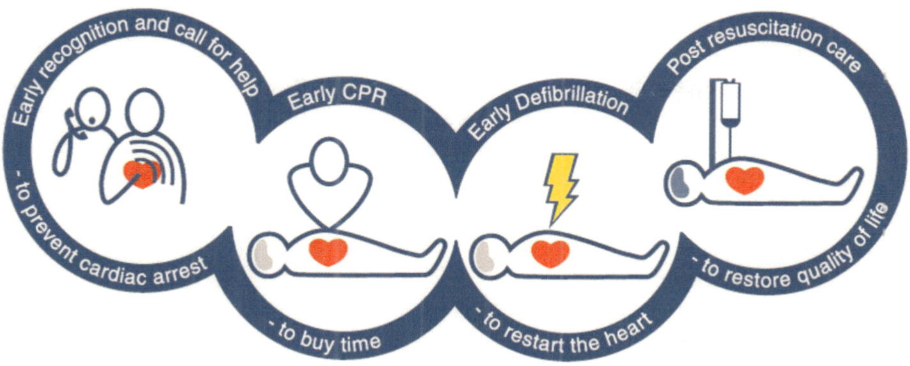

Figure 2.
The chain of survival [2].

The combination of both measures (early CPR and defibrillation) has a synergistic positive effect on outcome.

Different organizations around the world offer slightly different representations of the most important set of steps during resuscitation, known as "The Chain of Survival." Such sets of images have been created and are used to facilitate the perception of information and the necessary actions that should be taken by the first responder (early recognition, calling for help, bystander CPR, early defibrillation, emergency care by medical personnel, and postresuscitation care).

As soon as the AED is brought, the defibrillator should be turned on, and the electrode pads should be attached, placing them on the victim's chest (without clothes). If there is more than one rescuer, cardiopulmonary resuscitation is not interrupted during electrode placement. Next, follow the AED's spoken/visual instructions. Ensure no one touches the victim while the AED analyzes the heart rhythm. If defibrillation is indicated, ensure no one has touched the victim, press the discharge button as directed, and resume cardiopulmonary resuscitation immediately after repeated instructions. If defibrillation is not indicated, resume CPR immediately after heart rhythm analysis. Follow up on AED instructions.

If an AED is not available, continue CPR. Resuscitation measures are not stopped until a medical worker tells them to stop it, the victim confidently starts to wake up, moves and breathes normally, or the rescuer loses all strength.

The European Resuscitation Council and other organizations offer ""The Chain of Survival," which is a metaphorical representation of a series of critical actions that rescuers should take to improve the chances of survival after cardiac arrest (**Figure 2**).

Several studies conducted on cardiac arrest resuscitations have confirmed that the most important steps in the "chain of survival" are the early stages of the chain – timely recognition of cardiac arrest and initiation of CPR. Both of these are more often performed by nonmedical peers, so these people play an important role in further development. Knowing and understanding these links in the chain can reduce the mortality rate.

4. History and personalities

Personalities have influenced our ability to help people in critical situations involving spontaneous circulatory arrest related to ventricular fibrillation.

Peter Christian Abildgaard.

In 1775, the Danish veterinarian and doctor Peter Christian Abildgaard conducted experiments with electric countershock on animals. He managed to first kill the birds with an electric shock and then revive them with a countershock applied to the chest. Ventricular fibrillation and defibrillation were unknown and undocumented at this early date, but his report suggests that he made these changes long before other physiologists described them. Dr. Abildgar's long and varied career included many important contributions to veterinary and human medicine, biology, zoology, botany, physics, chemistry, and mineralogy.

Abildgaard founded the Christian Veterinary School in 1773, which is one of the oldest schools in Europe and whose first library contained Abildgaard's own collection. In 1858, the school was moved to Frederiksberg to become the Royal Veterinary and Agricultural University, and today it forms the Faculty of Natural Sciences of the University of Copenhagen.

Birth December 22, 1740 Copenhagen.

Death 21 January 1801 (aged 60) Copenhagen (**Figure 3**).

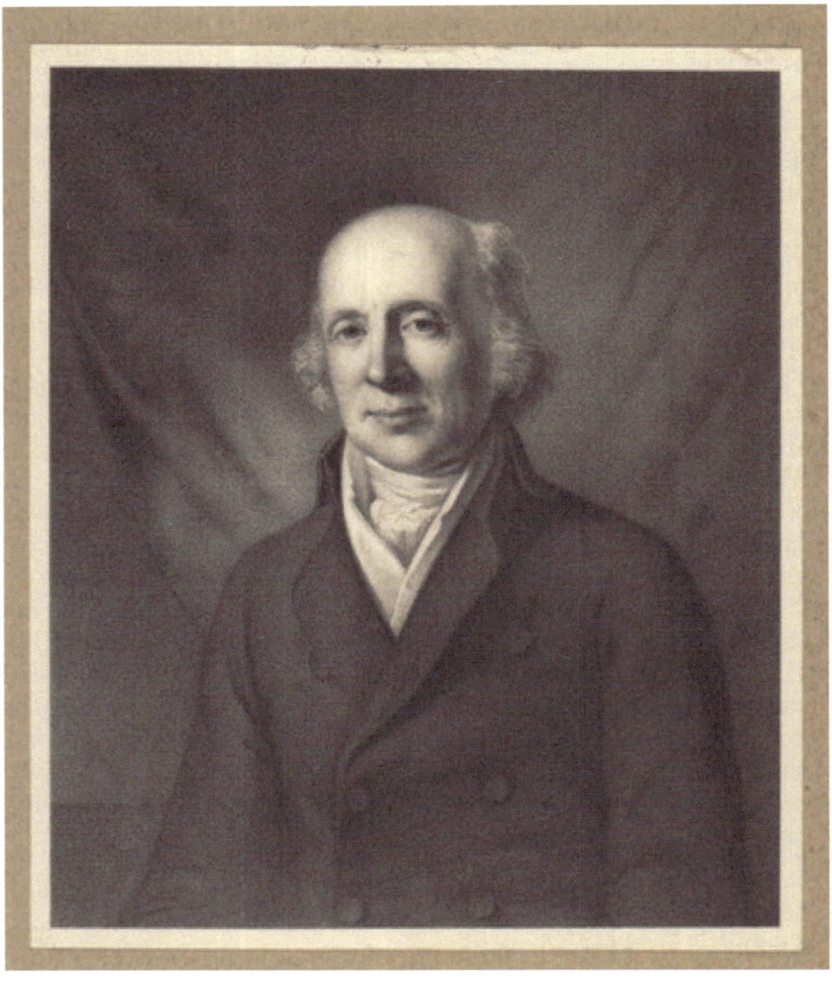

Figure 3.
***Peter Christian Abildgaard** [5].*

John Alexander McWilliam.

Professor John Alexander McWilliam of the University of Aberdeen was outstanding in the development and understanding of sudden death and the mechanisms of ventricular fibrillation. McWilliams studied the mechanisms of ventricular fibrillation and was the first scientist to link ventricular fibrillation to sudden death. He has a very important role in the research of arrhythmia mechanisms, McWilliams' works discussed the possibility of stopping ventricular fibrillation with an electric shock and also recommended transthoracic electrostimulation as a nontaxing treatment method in case of asystole. John McWilliams became a professor at the University of Aberdeen at the age of 29.

Born on July 31, 1857.

Died on January 13, 1937.

McWilliams' research on the physiology of ventricular fibrillation and sudden death, as well as the defined basic concepts, have remained relevant throughout the centuries and significantly influenced later scientific research and practice in clinical cardiology and electrophysiology, as well as served as a basis for the development of the basic principles of cardiopulmonary resuscitation. It was McWilliams who was the first scientist to develop the concept of ventricular fibrillation as a cause of sudden death. His methods are the basis of many modern clinical studies. The study of the role of the autonomic nervous system in modulating the electrical and mechanical properties of the heart began directly with the works of this scientist (**Figure 4**).

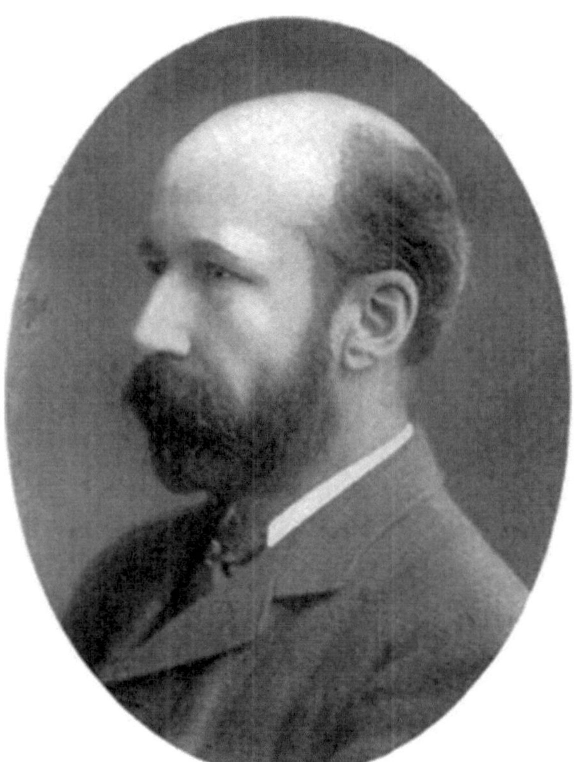

Figure 4.
***John Alexander McWilliam** [6].*

Albert Salisbury Hyman.

Cardiologist Albert Salisbury Hyman in the USA between 1930 and 1932, in cooperation with his brother Charles, created an interesting and, at that time, unseen electromechanical device, which was able to cause myocardial contractions with the help of electrical impulses. This Hyman invention can be called one of the first artificial pacemakers. One example of Hyman's heart "electric machine" is on display at the Heart Rhythm Society's museum. There are also reports in the literature about the use of this equipment in practice with experimental animals and there are data that the equipment was used to help at least one patient.

Born in 1893.

Died in 1972 (**Figures 5** and **6**).

In 1933, Popular Mechanics published an article about a new device developed by Dr. Albert Hyman and his brother Charles, an electrical research engineer. The device is described as a "Dead Man's Heart Self-Starting Device." The device can be compared to a car's automatic starter, because when the car's engine stops, the starter

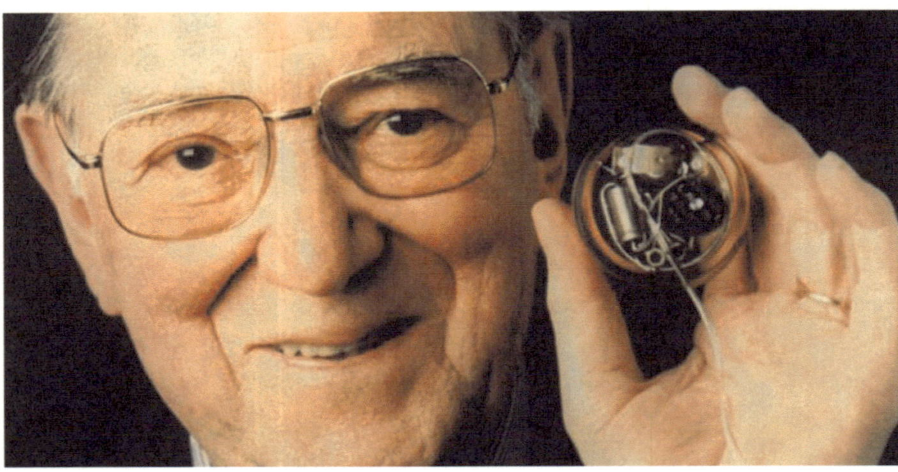

Figure 5.
Albert Salisbury Hyman *[7].*

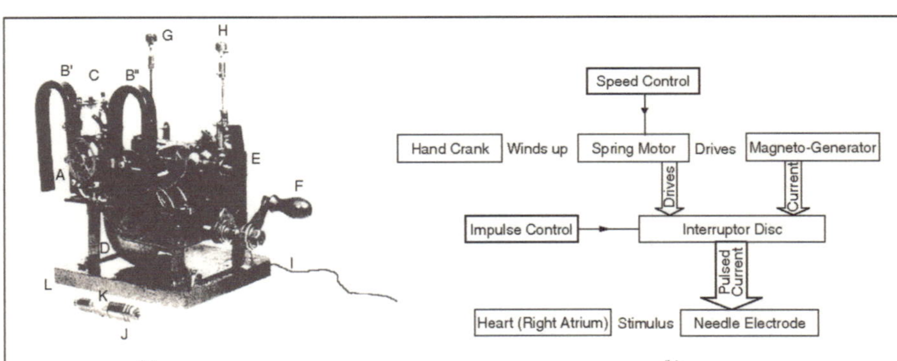

Figure 6.
Diagram and principle of operation of the first Hyman artificial pacemaker [8].

motor turns it over again until the cylinders start working again. In a similar way, the new device is able to give an electrical signal to the heart to start working again. In Albert Hyman's description, this was done by inserting one needle between the ribs and the other into the auricle of the right atrium of the heart, then starting the generator and turning it to the correct frequency. The article concludes that the medical establishment predicts widespread utility for the device, called the "Hyman Otor."

Mark C Lidwell.

Australian anesthesiologist Mark C. Lidwell first used the artificial heart pacemaker (the principle of this method and the equipment at his disposal) in clinical practice in a Sydney hospital as early as 1926, but in history, it is Hyman's name that is associated with the concept of "artificial pacemaker," which the medical and nonmedical community still used today. It is debatable who really deserves the laurels of the first discoverer, but Lidwell did not patent his device and chose to remain anonymous for many years. It is true, however, that in the medical circles of that time, the opinion against Hyman's version was quite contradictory, and it was not accepted in the professional environment for a long time (**Figure** 7).

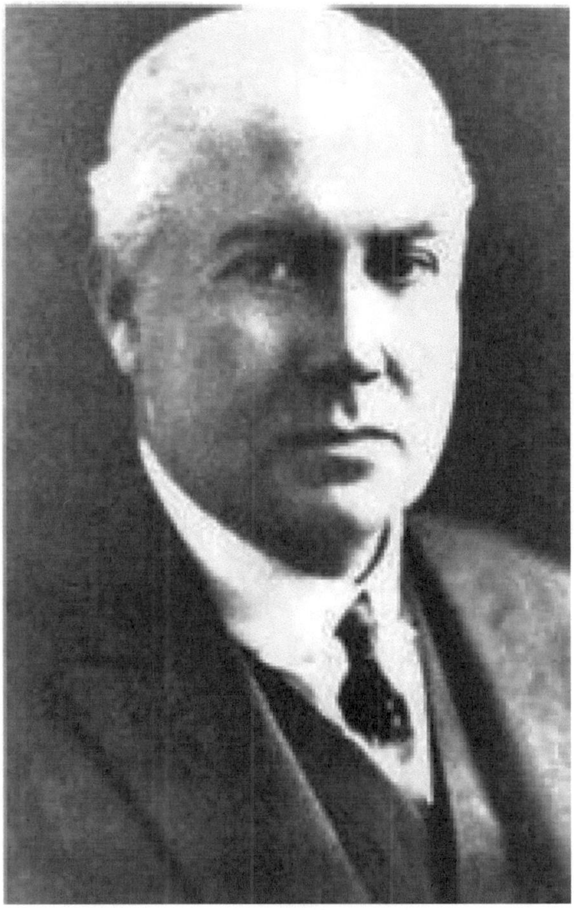

Figure 7.
Mark C Lidwell *(in some published and available sources mark C Lidwill) [9].*

Federico Battelli.

Federico Battelli (Italian Federico Battelli) or Frederic Battelli (Fr. Frédéric Battelli; April 6, 1867, Macerata Feltre; September 5, 1941, Geneva) was an Italian-Swiss physiologist and biochemist. Brother of Angelo Battelli.

He studied medicine in Urbino and Turin. In 1885, he began teaching at the Faculty of Medicine of the University of Turin, but then left Italy for political reasons and settled in Switzerland, taking a position as an assistant in the Physiology Department of the University of Geneva under Jean. -Louis Prevost, and in 1913 he succeeded his mentor as Professor of Physiology and held it until the end of his life.

Together with Prevost at the turn of the century, he studied death by electrocution and the effects of electricity on the heart muscle; these works anticipated later discoveries in the field of cardiac resuscitation. In 1909, together with L. S. Stern, he synthesized alcohol dehydrogenase for the first time.

Swiss physiologists Jean-Louis Prevost and Frédéric Batelli confirmed in 1899 that electric shocks can cause ventricular fibrillation in dogs, but even stronger shocks can stop the ventricular fibrillation and restore a normal physiological rhythm (**Figure 8**).

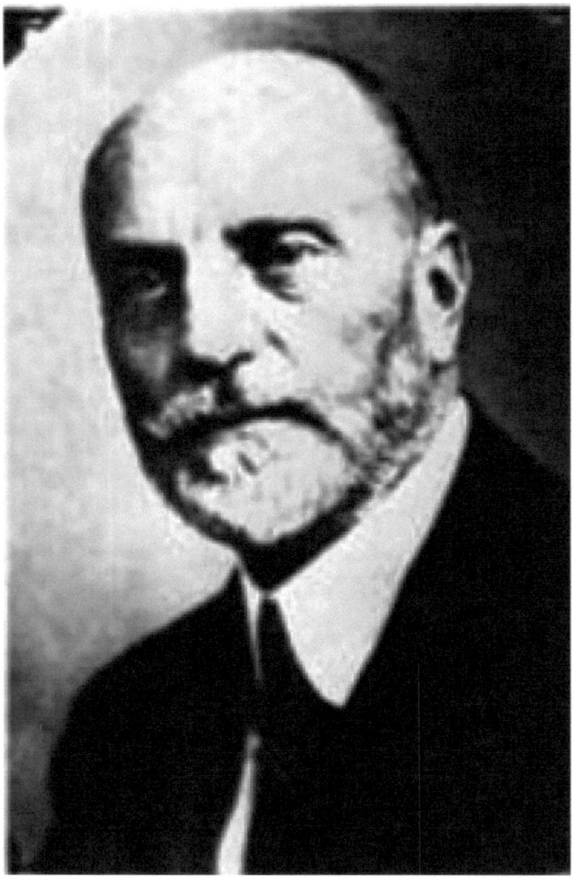

Figure 8.
***Federico Battelli** [10].*

William Bennett Kouwenhoven.

William Bennett Kouwenhoven is often called the father of cardiopulmonary resuscitation in the professional environment, and this is not a mistake. Interestingly, Kouwenhoven began his professional and scientific career with a doctorate in engineering at the Technical University of Karlsruhe, Germany, and later moved to Baltimore, USA, to Johns Hopkins University, where he worked both as a scientist and as a dean, in cooperation with the Edison Electrical Institute and the support of the same J. Hopkins University School of Medicine, he and his colleagues managed to develop a real-life defibrillator that can be applied to a closed chest. This scientist has outstanding merits in introducing the closed chest compression method into resuscitation practice. Kovenhoven has received many major awards, including the Albert Lasker Award for Research in Clinical Medicine and an honorary doctorate from Johns Hopkins University.

Born on January 13, 1886.

Died on November 10, 1975 (**Figure 9**).

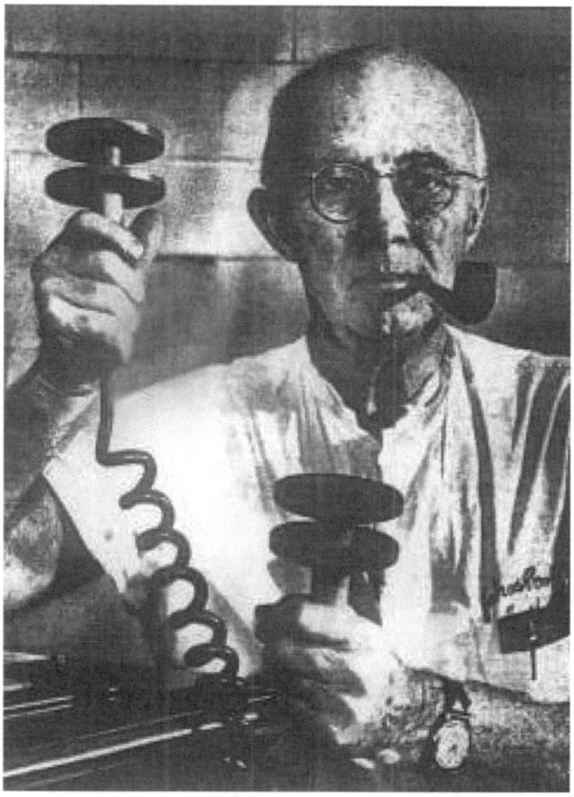

Figure 9.
***William Bennett Kouwenhoven** [11].*

Claude Schaeffer Beck.

Claude Schaefer Beck has left many records for himself in history. He was also a candidate for the Nobel Prize in Medicine in 1952. Throughout his career, Beck has always been an advocate and supporter of highly innovative methods. Beck's operations are still methodologically recognized, cardiopericardiopexy (Beck's operation I) in 1935 and the creation of a shunt between the aorta and coronary sinus (Beck's operation II) in 1940 can be found in any medical textbooks and are still appreciated by the specialist community. The pectoral muscle implantation technique in the

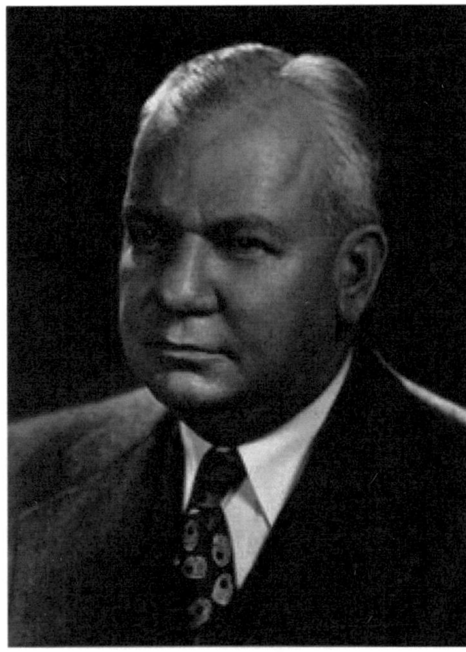

Figure 10.
Claude Schaeffer Beck [10, 12].

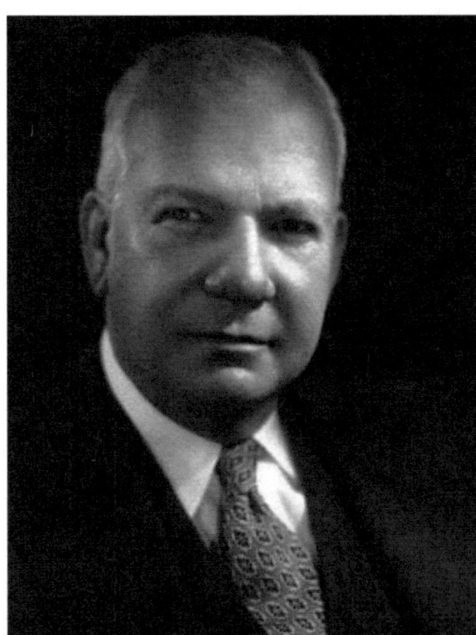

Figure 11.
Claude Schaeffer Beck [10, 12].

pericardium, which was performed by Beck back in 1930, which was a very innovative method for those times, has lost its relevance today, but at that time was very well received in the professional environment.

In terms of resuscitation, Beck's name is associated with the successful defibrillation during surgery of a 14-year-old boy with congenital heart defects who went into cardiac arrest after surgery. After 45 minutes of ineffective direct (manual) heart massage after repeated chest opening, Beck applied a defibrillator built by Rand Development Corp. and designed by Beck himself. A normal heartbeat was restored, and the boy made a full recovery.

Beck's name in clinical medicine is also associated with the analysis of the physiological basis of the signs of cardiac tamponade, and clinicians call these signs Beck's triad. The signs are low arterial blood pressure (hypotension), distended neck veins, and distant, muffled heart sounds.

Please do not confuse with Aaron Beck's triad, which is associated with depression.

Born on November 8, 1894.

Died on October 14, 1971 (**Figures 10** and **11**).

Paul Morris Zoll.

Paul Morris Zoll (July 15, 1911 to January 5, 1999) was a Jewish-American cardiologist and one of the pioneers of the artificial pacemaker and cardiac defibrillator. He graduated from Boston Latin School in 1928.

During his long professional career, Paul Zoll managed to divide his time equally between clinical work and scientific research. The results of his research led to a paradigm shift in the practice of cardiology. For example, the pacing of a stopped heart from the surface of the chest in 1952; monitoring of clinically significant cardiac

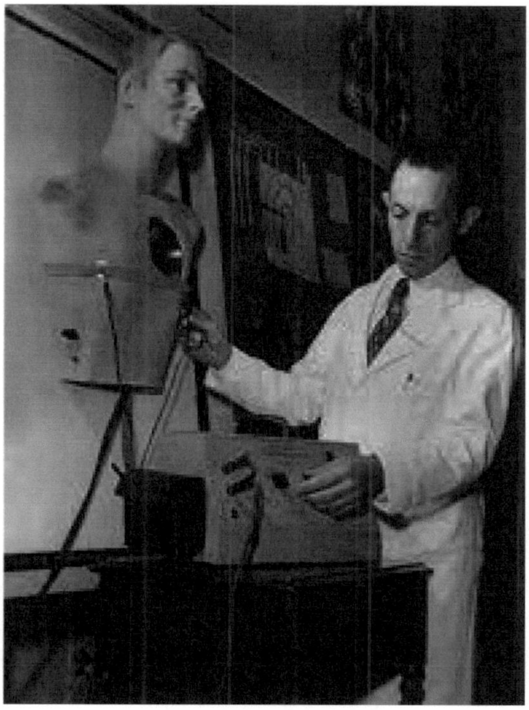

Figure 12.
Paul Morris Zoll [13].

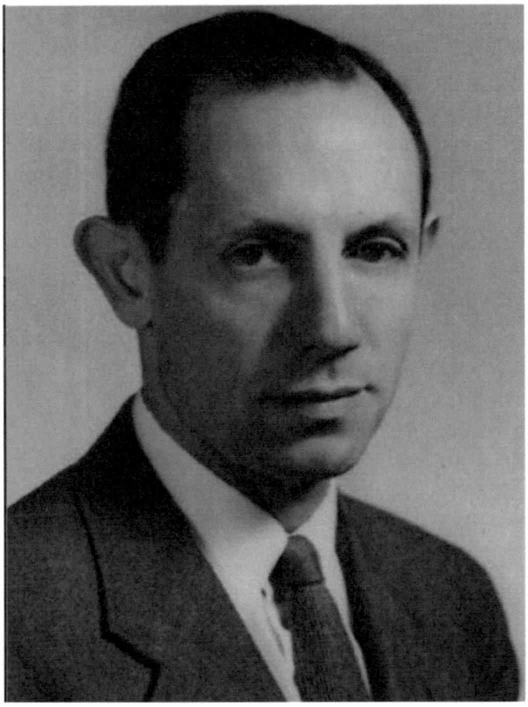

Figure 13.
Paul Morris Zoll [13].

arrhythmias in 1953; performing defibrillation from the chest surface to stop life-threatening ventricular fibrillation in 1956; Installation of a Zoll-Belgard-Electrodyne self-contained long-term pacemaker in a child in 1960; and the introduction of a new concept that allowed for "painless" electrostimulation of the chest surface in 1982. The new device led to the formation of a small company that later became known as Zoll Medical Corporation.

In collaboration with Alan Belgard, chief electrical engineer and co-owner of Electrodyne, effective chest surface pacemakers were developed to meet Paul Zoll's needs. This collaboration became long-lasting as they jointly developed a series of chest surface pacemakers (transthoracic), monitors for clinically significant heart rhythm disturbances, external defibrillators, cardiac monitors – automatic pacemakers, and long-term implantable pacemakers (**Figures 12** and **13**).

Bernard Lown.

Bernard Lown has many merits in the development of both electrophysiology and cardiosurgery, as well as in intensive care pharmacotherapy. Precisely in 1961, in an experimental way, Lown's group with his colleagues were able to prove that a special direct current waveform can stop the fibrillation process without causing damage to the skeletal muscles and myocardium. This, in the words of the authors, "low waveform," did not cause electrical injury to the muscle tissue and did not traumatically affect the conduction system of the heart. This discovery was a big step toward the development of defibrillators and their introduction around the world.

Lown's work significantly improved the survival of patients with coronary heart disease, both in acute situations, and also had a significant impact on outcomes during cardiosurgical operations using artificial blood circulation techniques. According to

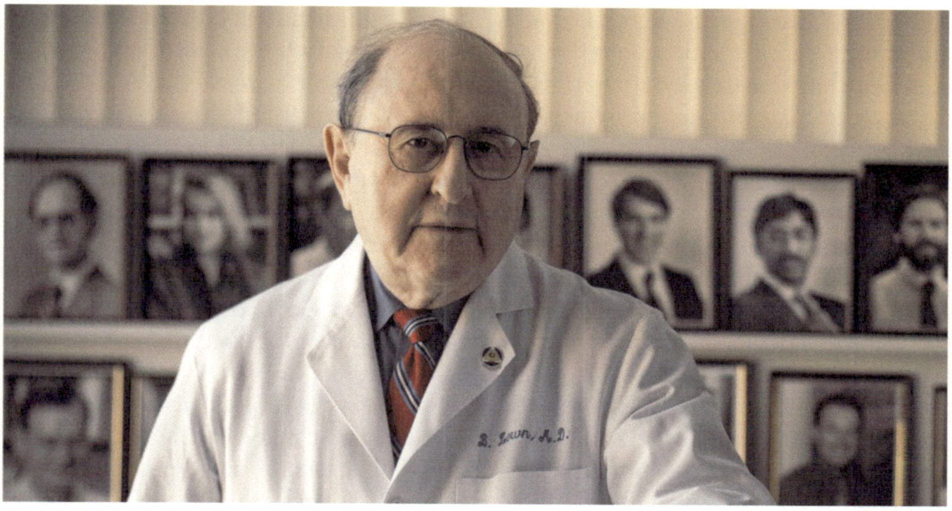

Figure 14.
Bernard Lown [14].

literature sources, in 1962, Donald B. Effler was the first cardiosurgeon, who performed the first coronary artery bypass surgery both in his own operations and later in the same hospital, René Favloro, in 1967, and purposefully used a defibrillator to restore a physiological heartbeat.

Lown's research also touched on the use of electrical discharges to terminate arrhythmias that were not directly life-threatening to patients. Since then, the term "electrical cardioversion" has been introduced into clinical practice.

In the field of pharmacotherapy, Lown's influence changed the attitude toward cardiac glycoside digitoxin, which until the 50s of the last century, was widely used for the treatment of congestive heart failure and often encountered the toxic effects of the drug. By replacing the long-acting digitoxin with the shorter-acting digoxin and additionally intensively controlling the potassium concentration, the patient's survival improved significantly. Lown studied the relationship between the concentration of potassium and the intensity of the use of diuretics and the correlations of the results and also introduced the drug lidocaine into the cardiology practice, which was previously only used as an anesthetic in the stomatology practice.

It is interesting that Bernards Lown was born in Utena, on the territory of Lithuania, in a family of Jews living in Lithuania, in 1935 he moved to the USA, New England state, Maine, where he started studying zoology at the University of Maine. He further developed his professional career in the USA in connection with the John Hopkins University School of Medicine, Yale University, New Haven, Connecticut, and the Peter Bent Brigham Hospital, now Brigham and Women's Hospital, in Boston. Lown was the founder of the Lown Cardiovascular Center and the Lown Cardiovascular Research Foundation.

Born on June 7, 1921.

Died on February 16, 2021 (**Figure 14**).

James Francis Pantridge.

James Francis Pantridge, CBE MC OStJ was a Northern Irish physician, cardiologist, and professor who transformed emergency medical and paramedic services with the invention of the portable defibrillator.

By 1957 Pantridge and his colleague Dr. John Geddes had introduced a modern cardiopulmonary resuscitation (CPR) system for the early treatment of cardiac arrest. Further research led Frank Pantridge to realize that many of the deaths were due to ventricular fibrillation, which should have been treated before the patient was admitted to the hospital. Analyzing and evaluating these facts, he created a system called Mobile Coronary Care (MCCU), an ambulance equipped with special equipment and appropriately trained personnel to provide specialized prehospital medical care.

Paintridge's outstanding contribution was the development of a portable defibrillator which was installed in a Belfast Ambulance Service vehicle. The first version of this device did not stand out with special portability and the ability to easily move it (weight around 70 kg and operated from a car battery), but in a short time until 1968, an excellent portable device was developed, which weighed 3 kg and which worked thanks to the miniature capacitor made by the National Aeronautics and Space Administration (NASA). When mentioning Paintridge, it would not be correct not to mention the engineer John Anderson, head of biomedical services at the Royal Victoria Hospital in Belfast, who later became a co-founder of Heartsine.

In 1967, an article was published in the Lancet magazine about these defibrillators and their role in saving people's lives. The Belfast system of treatment and management of emergency critical, life-threatening situations was

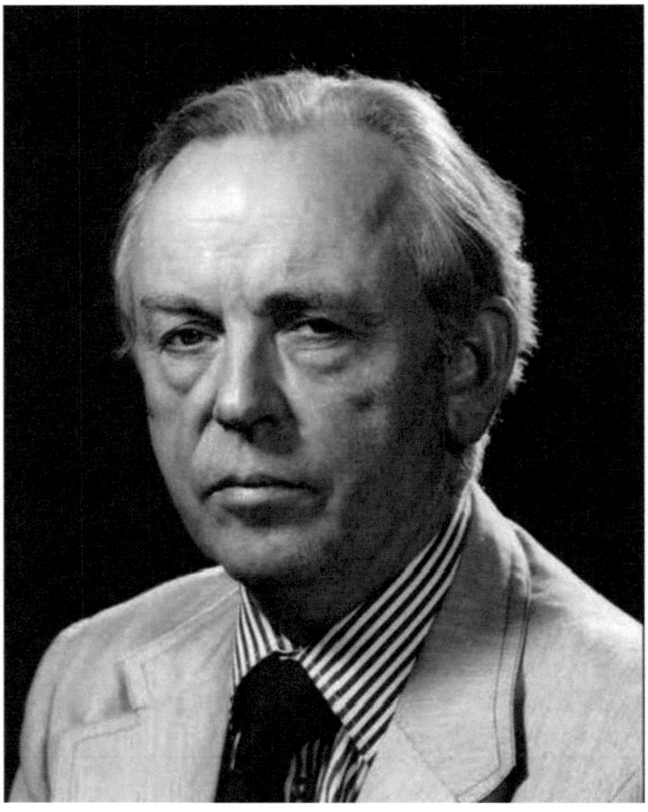

Figure 15.
James Francis Pantridge [15].

accepted by emergency services around the world, often referred to professionally as the Paintridge Plan. The portable or portable defibrillator was recognized as the main means of first aid in life-critical situations, and the developed automated external defibrillator allowed it to be safely recommended for use even by nonspecialists in emergency situations.

As strange as it may seem, James Francis Pantridge, who is known worldwide as the "father of emergency medicine," was little known in his country for a long time. It was not until after 1990 that all ambulances in the UK were equipped with portable defibrillators.

Born on October 3, 1916.

Died on December 26, 2004 (**Figure 15**).

Barouh Vojtec Berkovits.

Barouh Vojtec Berkovits (May 7, 1926 to October 23, 2012 [16]) was one of the pioneers of bioengineering, especially the cardiac defibrillator and artificial cardiac pacemaker. In particular, Berkowitz invented the "demand pacemaker" and the direct current defibrillator.

Berkovits was born in Czechoslovakia. He immigrated to the United States in the 1950s and worked for the pacemaker company Medtronic from 1975 until his retirement. In 1982, Berkovits received the Heart Rhythm Society's "Outstanding Scientist Award." Graduated from New York University's Tandon School of Engineering in 1956. He was also a faculty member at NYU Tandon (**Figure 16**).

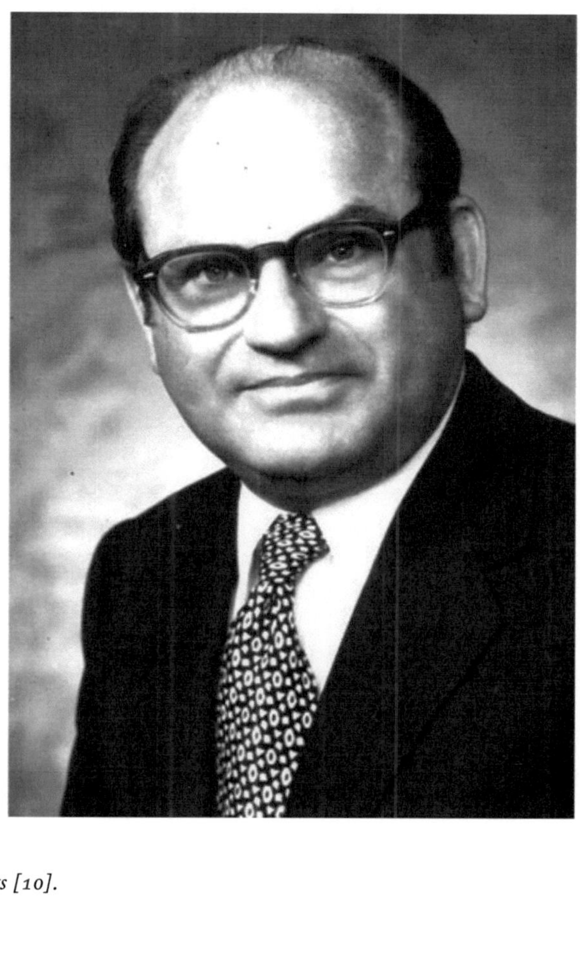

Figure 16.
Barouh Vojtec Berkovits [10].

Carl John Wiggers.

Carl John Wiggers (May 28, 1883 to April 28, 1963) was a physician and medical researcher famous for his research on the heart and blood pressure.

Wiggers' main merits are associated with the discovery and implementation of a new method to be able to record the activity of the heart together with the blood pressure of different stages, as well as the effect of low oxygenation on the activity of the heart. Wiggers has outstanding merits in the study of the impact of shock effects, in the study of the impact of heart valve defects on heart function. Two excellent medical experts, scientists – Carl John Wiggers and Claude Beck together created the excellent Wiggers diagram, which is still used in the teaching process of students and doctors when we talk about the physiology of the cardiovascular system.

Carl John Wiegers is the first editor of the renowned medical journal Circulation Research, has written seven books, and is the author of more than 300 scientific articles. In 1952, he received the Golden Heart Award from the American Heart Association. In 1951, he was elected to the National Academy of Sciences. Wigers was awarded the highly prestigious Modern Medicine Award in 1954 and the Albert Lasker Award in 1955 for outstanding achievements in cardiovascular research.

From 1918 to 1953, Carl John Wiegers was Professor and Chairman of the Department of Physiology at Western Reserve University School of Medicine, which became known as Case Western Reserve University School of Medicine (**Figures 17** and **18**).

In 1940, together with Dr. René Wegria (Dr. René Wegria, College of Physicians and Surgeons, Columbia University) discovered that ventricular fibrillation can be induced during a precise period called the "vulnerable period." From these studies, the science of the cardiac pacemaker of the future was concluded [19].

4.1 Defibrillators

The development of defibrillators used in practical everyday medicine began in the twentieth century and is already in the 20s. As the availability of technical

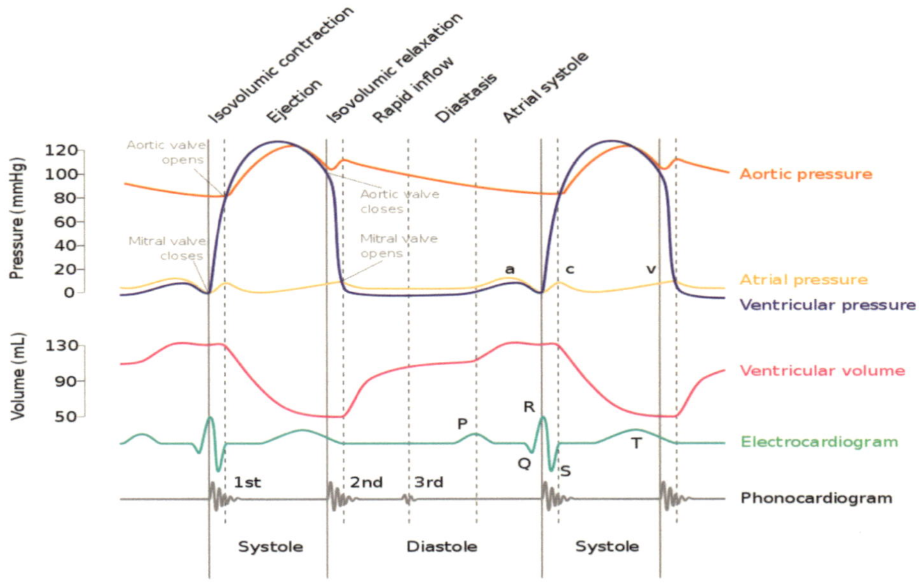

Figure 17.
Wiggers diagram [17].

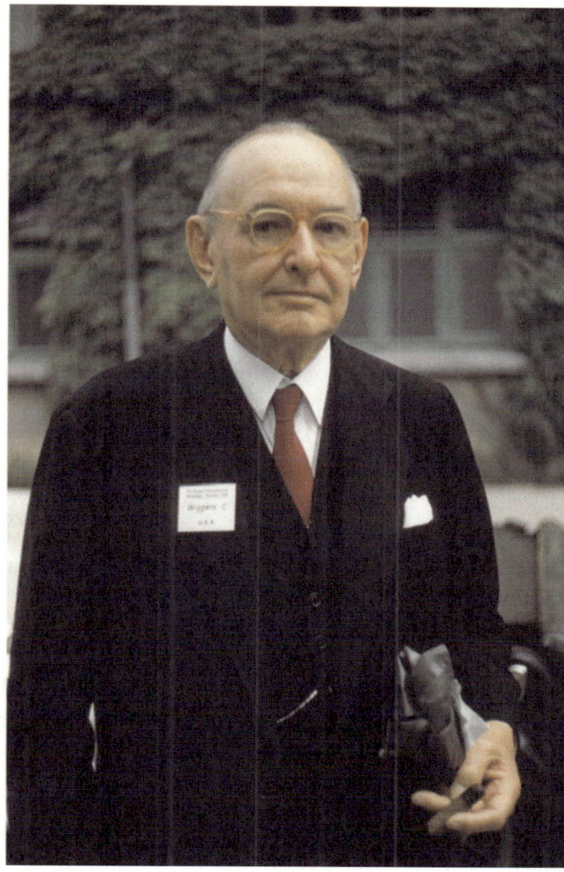

Figure 18.
Carl John Wiggers [18].

achievements increased and, first of all, the use of electricity in everyday life, the number of electrocutions began to increase. People's lifestyles and standards have also changed their views on the possibilities of providing emergency care on an ever-widening scale. Substantial support for these programs was provided by Consolidated Edison of New York by establishing a cooperative project and supporting research with funding. We have already mentioned Beck's defibrillation during surgery, in which this methodology was used to revive a 14-year-old boy. Zoll, in 1956, reported the first successful application of the defibrillation method using external defibrillation. Technical parameters included 15 amperes of alternating current, which generated 710 volts, which were acquired in a transthoracic approach in 0.15 seconds (150 milliseconds). Alexander, Kleiger, and Lown first published in the literature the use of alternating current with the intention of terminating ventricular tachycardia (VT). In the publications of the beginning of the 60s, in the already mentioned publications of Alexander, Kleiger, and Lown, the superiority of direct current over alternating current was confirmed from the point of view of safety.

In the previous chapters, it was already mentioned that the first successful out-of-hospital defibrillation was performed in Belfast by the doctors of the emergency medical service of this city [20] Defibrillation was performed for the first time in Portland,

Oregon, USA for 1969, without the presence of doctors, when the procedure was performed by paramedics (paramedics) during an emergency. It was reported in 1972.

4.2 The beginnings of automatic defibrillators

At the beginning of the 70s in the state of Portland, doctors Arch Diak, W. Stanley Welborn and Robert Rulmen began to focus in depth on the development of AED prototypes [21]. Their work led to the creation of the Cardiac Resuscitator Corporation.

The work with the Heart Aid system in Brighton, UK, is usually cited as the first nonhospital trial in this context. The work started in 1980. Early prototypes weighed 28 pounds. Two electrodes were used to ensure their operation: an anterior thoracic electrode located on the chest to record ECG leads and sequentially record heart activity, as well as a second electrode located orally, or more precisely, orally/epigastrically, and deliver electric shocks as needed. This device was also able to stimulate the heart if necessary (known as transcutaneous or transthoracic electrical stimulation). In 1982, the US Food and Drug Administration (FDA) approved clinical trials of EMT defibrillation (EMT-D). The first US initiatives for this application of emergency medical techniques and defibrillation were in Washington, Iowa, Minnesota, and Tennessee.

In the early 1990s, successful training and use of AEDs by police officers and other first responders was reported. The FDA approved the lay use of AEDs in the 1990s, and Good Samaritan legislation soon followed. It could be said that the road to AED seemed to be clear and with green lights; however, several problems appeared over time. Some are quite serious and essential.

4.3 The nuances of operation of automatic external defibrillators

In the first AED models, in order to achieve the desired effect and obtain information about the heart's activity, relatively complex manipulations had to be performed when the AED was started. In situations where time is limited and every second is worth its weight in gold, this behavior prolonged the performance of adequate resuscitation. To achieve the required result, the oral/epigastric electrode had to be inserted first and the other electrode placed on the front of the patient's chest. AEDs in use today require the defibrillator electrodes to be placed on the right side of the chest and in the projection of the apex of the heart or on the front and back of the torso (this procedure applies to infants and young children). Electrodes serve both for heart rate monitoring and defibrillation. An AED can also notify the user when there is insufficient electrode contact, signal when the device is preparing for defibrillation, record and notify the responders when the patient's pulse should be checked, allow for recording when a nonshockable rhythm is present or when any spontaneous movement is detected.

4.4 Algorithms and possibilities of rhythm analysis

Early AED diagnostic algorithms were designed to respond primarily to a heart rate (usually ventricular rate) greater than 150 electrical complexes per minute (essentially electrical complexes) and an electrocardiographic QRS complex amplitude greater than 0.15 mm. Modern AED machines use a combined sum of several criteria to analyze the ECG rhythm. In addition to the previously applied frequency and QRS amplitude criteria, QRS data are analyzed in relation to its slope, complex morphology, power spectral density, and the time the complex is away from predefined isoelectric line levels, which in turn are defined as pathological. The device performs these checks at intervals of 2 to 4 seconds. The standard algorithm provides that if three consecutive parameter checks detect abnormal complexes with an intensity of occurrence at least twice as frequent as the QRS generated by any other site, the AED will be signaled to perform defibrillation.

Short-wave ventricular fibrillation (VF) is significantly more problematic than long-wave VF. Modern AEDs have special programs that allow you to make correlations and diagnostic compromises between setting the amplitude criterion with a sufficiently low sensitivity threshold. This shriek is low enough to recognize microwave ventricular fibrillation but maintains a sufficient threshold to not respond to asystole or artifacts. There are data in the literature that confirm that the sensitivity of VF detection of modern AED systems is 76–96%, but at the same time the specificity (correct detection of nonfibrillator rhythms) is close to 100%. In any case, considering the importance of AED and the real application environment as well as users, these features are extremely important.

4.5 Application of two-phase versus single-phase discharge

Monophasic defibrillation delivers electrical shock in one direction only. Biphasic defibrillation provides an electrical discharge in one direction for half of the discharge time and an electrical discharge in the opposite direction for the second half of the discharge.

Studies in dogs have shown less cardiac conduction disturbances and fewer ST-segment changes after biphasic electrical discharge than monophasic discharge. In clinical studies, it has been confirmed that monophasic electrical discharge is equivalent to biphasic discharge in cases of ventricular fibrillation induced by electrophysiological examinations. There are also similar data on the use of defibrillation techniques in the prehospital stage in patients with ventricular fibrillation and ventricular tachycardia. Research data shows that a biphasic waveform of 115 J is equivalent to a monophasic discharge waveform of approximately 200 J. Due to reduced discharge energy, virtually all implantable cardioverter-defibrillators (ICDs) use biphasic waveforms. Most AED manufacturers are switching to biphasic discharge technology, as the lower amount of energy used can result in both longer battery life and a shorter time to full charge.

Although the use of biphasic defibrillation may have theoretical clinical advantages, most patient studies, and reports have shown equivalence rather than the superiority of one form at equivalent doses (biphasic doses are lower).

4.6 Some important nuances need to be known when dealing with an AED

Most manufacturers recommend testing the AED at specified time intervals. Some devices need to be turned on to perform a self-test; other models have a built-in self-test system with a visible indicator that indicates the state of the battery and possible operation.

All manufacturers label their AED's pads with an expiration date, and it is important to ensure that AED defibrillation pads are within the appropriate expiration date. AED pads have a typical life expectancy of 18 to 30 months. Usually, these data are visible and on the outer side of the package. For many modern AED models, this date is visible through a "window" embedded in the body of the device, which, of course, facilitates their control and possible regular maintenance or replacement of equipment accessories. For some devices, however, you have to open the device case to make sure of the expiration dates. Logically, AEDs that are less complicated and simpler to maintain and control are preferred.

It is very important to make sure that the batteries in the AED device have not expired. The AED manufacturer will specify how often the batteries should be changed. Each AED has a different recommended maintenance schedule outlined in the user manual. Each AED has a specific checklist that includes a monthly battery capacity check, including checking the green indicator light when it is on, the condition and cleanliness of all cables and the device, and checking that there is enough power to perform the defibrillation procedure in sufficient time in number.

When the AED is turned on, or the case (box) of the device is opened, it will automatically prompt the user to attach the electrodes (pads) to the patient (the latest models are provided with a voice command system, which may be adapted to different countries with different basic languages). When the defibrillation pads are attached, everyone should avoid touching the patient to avoid false device readings. The pads allow the AED to check the electrical signals from the heart and determine if the patient is in a shockable rhythm (ventricular fibrillation or ventricular tachycardia). If the device detects that an appropriate situation exists and a defibrillation shock is necessary, it will use the battery to charge its internal capacitor in preparation for delivering an electric shock. The system of the device is safe enough – charging and preparation for defibrillation are done only when necessary.

Once the device has charged its system, it tells the user (usually with a loud beep) that no one touches the patient and then tells them to press a button to deliver the electrical discharge; The standard requires human intervention to deliver a defibrillation shock (by pressing a button) to avoid accidental shock injury to another person (which may occur in response to the patient or a bystander touching the patient at the time of the shock), as AEDs are expected to be used in public areas, often in a limited space, and the public response in such extreme situations is not always predictable. Many modern models will automatically analyze the patient's heartbeat according to the built-in algorithm after an electric shock and will either order CPR or prepare for the next shock.

Many AEDs have a special feature called "event memory" that stores the patient's ECG, as well as all the information obtained regarding the time the device was activated, the number of shocks delivered, and the strength of those shocks. A voice recording option exists for several equipment groups [22] in order to be able to analyze the actions taken by the medical staff and to be able to analyze whether these actions have an impact on the performance results, respectively, on survival. The material recorded in the device system can be used both in the recording of computer systems and also made available in another format (printed, graphically) so that the assisting organization, professional association, or government bodies can analyze the effect of CPR and defibrillation on survival. Some AEDs are able to collect data on the resuscitation process and to assess the quality of chest compressions.

Unlike conventional defibrillators, using an automated external defibrillator (AED) requires only minimal basic training, or some AED versions allow you to do it without any skills at all. This possibility is provided by a special sound information system, or so-called "electronic voice" that tells the helper every next step of the operation.

Such AEDs are approved for use in the United States and many other countries. Given that the responder may be hearing impaired or unable to fully understand the language in which the AED provides information, most modern AEDs also have special visual instructions with special pictograms. The placement of AEDs in public and freely accessible places, as well as the ease of their use, has created the concept of public access defibrillation (PAD). It should be noted that most often the first persons who start resuscitation are not specially trained people or professional doctors.

One of the most important functions of an AED is the ability to record and automatically detect a heart rhythm and, guided by the recorded data, automatically determine whether a shock should be delivered. In practice, fully automatic models are used, which are able to carry out an electric discharge even without the helper's command. Semi-automatic models will tell the user that a shock is needed, but the user must tell the machine, usually by pressing a button. In most cases, the user cannot ignore the AED's "no shock" warning. Some AEDs can be used on children who weigh less than 55 pounds (25 kg) or who are younger than 8 years old. If a specific AED model is approved for pediatric use, only more suitable pads should be used.

4.7 Benefits of AEDs

Clinical studies confirm that public access defibrillators (PADs), when available and used correctly during out-of-hospital cardiac arrest, were associated with a 40% median survival rate. Even in situations where they are handled by nonspecialists without training, sudden death victims have a much higher chance of survival. It should be noted that in many publicly accessible AED locations, the device's location block is linked to the emergency medical system or rescue services dispatch office. An alarm signal is immediately received, and professionals immediately rush to the rescue.

5. Classic AED studies

5.1 Location

Classic AED studies have examined the effectiveness of AEDs in urban, suburban, and rural settings.

Seattle.

In 1987, Cummins et al. reported a controlled trial comparing the effectiveness of AEDs with manual defibrillators used by EMTs to treat 147 patients with ventricular fibrillation (VF) in suburban Seattle, Washington. No statistically significant differences were observed in admission rates (54% AED; 50% manual) or survival to discharge (30% AED; 23% manual [23].

In 1988, Weaver et al. reported the results of AED practice by non-EMT first responders (event response time 3.3 minutes) compared to baseline CPR by first responders (event response time 3.4 minutes). This was followed by the involvement of paramedics with the application of an AED (response time to the event was 5.1 minutes). It is important to note that the AED model used was modified during the study. Overall results for the group of patients with ventricular fibrillation detected (504 patients) showed no significant difference in clinical parameters when assessing hospitalization (59% first responders, laypersons with AEDs; 53% professional paramedics with AEDs) but significantly higher patient survival and consecutive discharge from the hospital was observed in the first group of patients, those who had CPR with an AED administered by first responders (30% vs. 19%). Admission rate and discharge rate are not the same thing. [24]

Iowa.

In 1986, Stults et al. reported a study in a rural setting comparing AEDs with manual defibrillators used by EMTs. Results for 88 VF patients showed no significant difference in admission rates (29% AED; 32% manual) or survival to discharge (17% AED; 13% manual) [25].

Minnesota.

Bachmann et al. failed to confirm results from Iowa and Seattle in rural northeastern Minnesota [22]. They reported a survival-to-discharge rate of 11% for paramedics, 5% for EMTs with manual defibrillators, and 2.5% for cardiac arrests performed by EMTs performing CPR. A separate analysis of VF was not performed. They found no survivors of witness arrest, as had been the case in previous studies, and the results led them to question the use of AEDs in rural areas.

In contrast, Vukow studied EMT defibrillation in rural southeastern Minnesota in 1988 [26]. In a report of 63 patients, patients treated by EMTs with AEDs had significantly higher admission rates (30 vs. 12%) and survival to discharge (17 vs. 4%) than patients treated with EMT without AED.

Detroit, Chicago, and New York.

Reflections and also discussions were caused by the data presented by Detroit colleagues on the affectivity of revitalization. A total of 595 patients with circulatory arrest (cardiac arrest) of various causes underwent basic EMTs with AED application. The first finding confirmed that only 20% of these patients recorded VF. About 5% were hospitalized in a clinical condition defined as "alive," but none of these 5% were discharged alive. Analyzing such unpleasant results, it was concluded that the EMS response time exceeded 10 minutes, as well as the time from the event to the activation of the EMS system. It should be kept in mind that time is both the viability of the myocardium and the brain, as well as potential electrical activity in the myocardium. Unfortunately, this data was not published.

Similar studies reported a 4% survival rate from VF in Chicago and a 5% survival rate in New York. The average response time was more than 10–12 minutes.

Defibrillation "time to shock" analysis.

In the initial research conducted in Seattle, another interesting nuance was found: a significant time difference was recorded in the period until the defibrillation discharge was performed. AED defibrillation time was 1.1 minutes compared to 2 minutes for manual defibrillators. Bock and colleagues found that EMTs who used fully automated defibrillators on the job were, on average, 30 seconds faster in delivering shocks than their colleagues who used semi-automated devices [27].

AED Selection Factors Population density: Stapczynski et al. concluded that areas with population densities of less than 100 persons per square mile have minimal benefit from AEDs [28]. A study in Washington identified 172 sites with a much higher density of individuals (out of 71,000 sites). Similar local assessments, in conjunction with data analysis of emergency medical systems, can assist in the effective location of public AEDs. Increasingly, the placement of AEDs is more and more often directly related to places where there is an intense movement of people in intensive traffic nodes with a corresponding density of people in their location, which is more precisely depicted in the concept of public access defibrillation. Such places are airports, stadiums, large shopping malls, concert halls, and other places of mass events. The first airline to equip its transcontinental aircraft with AEDs (with an emphasis on transoceanic flights) was American Airlines in 1997. Subsequently, subsequent FAA regulations very quickly established the level of strict regulation that commercial passenger aircraft must be equipped with an AED and that aircraft personnel on board in their professional duties must be trained in the use of an AED (Aviation Medical Assistance Act of 1998, Section 121. part amendment). The reaction time was also regulated: the average reaction time to the AED application should be less than 4–6 minutes because only under this condition can a real positive effect from the AED be expected. Delta Airways, the Brazilian airline VARIG (also known as the VARIG study), and others were involved in the further implementation of AED in aviation. Currently, AEDs are the norm on any commercial flight. Levels of response systems: Multi-level response systems must be compatible equipment. If an AED is to be used by a first responder, the defibrillators or their electrode lead system must be compatible with the transport units listed below. Monitoring function: If the unit is also used by paramedics to monitor the patient's condition and not just by the AED technician in case of cardiac arrest, a monitor screen is required. Print options are also desirable.

Public access defibrillation.

Public access defibrillation (PAD) has been shown to be an important part of a successful chain of survival program [1]. AED placement has been most cost-effective in certain locations, including casinos, airports, stadiums, health clubs, universities, and senior centers [29–31].

A systematic review of AED availability and survival rates for out-of-hospital cardiac arrest, which included 16 studies with 55,537 participants, found that the one-month survival rate in schools, sports venues, and airports was 39.3% compared with 23.5% elsewhere. The 1-month survival rate was 39.3% in schools, sports venues, and airports, compared to 23.5% in other locations. Longer time between cardiac arrest and AED arrival and greater distance between AED location and cardiac arrest location were negatively correlated with one-month survival rates, but the correlations were not statistically significant [32].

5.2 Experiences and conclusions of some countries

Poland.

Zuratynski P. et al. performed an analysis of the use of AEDs, evaluating the frequency of their operation by calendar days, months of the year, seasonality, as well as time of day. It is interesting that AEDs were most often used in April and least often in November, and compared to the days of the week, AEDs were most often used on Fridays but less often on Sundays. More frequent out-of-hospital cardiac arrest (OHCA) events were noted between 12:00 and 16:00 during the day. If the day is divided into two stages: daytime 8:00–20:00 and nighttime 20:00–8:00, then the ratio of daytime and nighttime is 70–30%. [33]

Denmark.

According to the Register of Danish colleagues in the Danish capital, Copenhagen, the vast majority of AEDs were freely available during the day on all days of the week, but another very significant problem was their availability within 24 hours. 50 AEDs (9.1%) of all AEDs recorded in the public access system were available 24 hours a day, 7 days a week [34]. At the same time, we cannot fail to mention Lin Zhang et al., the

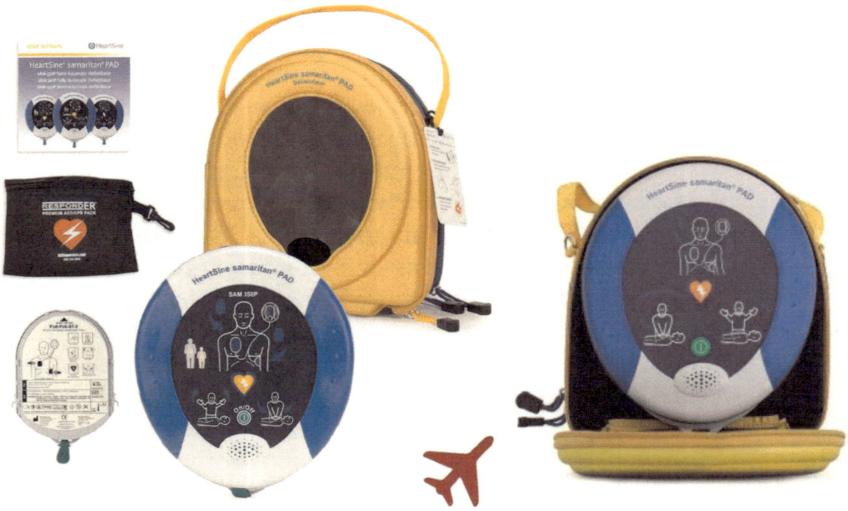

Figure 19.
Automatic external defibrillator [37].

very important sentence indicated in the publication about 40% of AEDs registered in three districts of Shanghai, which are located in school buildings or government institutions, and their availability restrictions are related to security concerns [35]. Full public availability of AEDs has also been noted as a problem in Toronto, Canada, and many other cities. Some AEDs are located in large office buildings, institutions, supermarkets, universities, and schools, which are closed in the evening hours, and some of them are also on holidays; sequentially, AEDs are theoretically available, but practically there is no possibility to use them in practice. Similar problems with AED availability within 24 hours and throughout the week were demonstrated by Agerskova et al. In the OHCA analysis in Copenhagen [36].

Thirty-day survival in people after OHCA almost doubled in cases where the event was in a location where the nearest AED was within 200 m of the scene. This concept is also used in planning the placement of AEDs in grandstands of large stadiums, shopping malls, concert halls, and similar mass gathering places.

Mortality after OHCA is significantly influenced by time: both the time in which CPR is started and, even more, the time how quickly an AED can be used to save the patient's life. Public access to defibrillators and their location information – key solutions to improve survival (**Figure 19**).

6. Instead of an afterword

This chapter is only a small part of the interesting world that opens up when you start to delve into the nuances of resuscitation and the problems associated with it, as well as the history of this medical field. Not infrequently, the pioneers of the field have had to overcome a wall of profound opposition and misunderstanding, but in the end, science has won, and all of us, the medical profession, the people associated with it, and those whom this knowledge and discoveries have helped to return to this side of the River Styx, are grateful, to the great minds who contributed to the progress of medicine.

DOI: http://dx.doi.org/10.5772/intechopen.112518

Automated external defibrillators are an excellent example of collaboration between medicine, biology, and engineering. The authors of this chapter each have their own experience and resuscitated patients, one in intensive care cardiology, another in the emergency medicine system, and another also during veteran basketball competitions. How great it is if you have this great and seemingly invisible helper nearby or even next to you – an AED. And how many lives he has helped save and how many more he will help, together with our professional knowledge and skill.

Author details

Oskars Kalejs[1*], Aija Maca-Kaleja[1], Ketija Apsite[1], Anita Abula[1] and Laura Strazdina[2]

1 Riga Stradins University, P. Stradins Clinical University Hospital, Latvia

2 Turiba University, Latvia

*Address all correspondence to: okalejs@gmail.com

IntechOpen

© 2023 The Author(s). Licensee IntechOpen. This chapter is distributed under the terms of the Creative Commons Attribution License (http://creativecommons.org/licenses/by/3.0), which permits unrestricted use, distribution, and reproduction in any medium, provided the original work is properly cited.

References

[1] Ringh M, Hollenberg J, Palsgaard-Moeller T, et al. The challenges and possibilities of public access defibrillation. Journal of Internal Medicine. 2018;**283**(3):238-256

[2] Perkins GD, Handley AJ, Koster KW, Castren M, Smyth M, Olasveengen T, et al. European resuscitation council guidelines for resuscitation 2015 section 2. Adult basic life support and automated external defibrillation. Resuscitation. 2015;**95**:81-99

[3] Sudden cardiac arrest. Mayoclinic. December 28.12.2019. Available from: https://www.mayoclinic.org/diseases-conditions/sudden-cardiac-arrest/symptoms-causes/syc-20350634

[4] Podrid PJ. Overview of sudden cardiac arrest and sudden cardiac death. UpToDate. August 2019. Available from: https://www-uptodate-com.db.rsu.lv/contents/overview-of-sudden-cardiac-arrest-and-https://www.uptodate.com/contents/overview-of-sudden-cardiac-arrest-and-sudden-cardiac-death

[5] Abildgaard PC. Available from: http://www5.kb.dk/images/billed/2010/okt/billeder/object148390/en

[6] McWillam History. 02.07.2012. Available from: http://mcwhistory.blogspot.com/2012/07/prof-john-alexander-macwilliam.html

[7] Episode 14 – The invention of the pacemaker (cardiostimulator). Available from: http://icardio.ca/en/articles/history-of-cardiology/the-invention-of-the-pacemaker-cariostimulator

[8] Haddad SA, Houben R, Serdijin WA. The evolution of pacemakers. IEEE Engineering in Medicine and Biology Magazine. 2006;**25**(3):38-48

[9] Mond HG, Wickha GG, Sloman JG. The Australian history of cardiac pacing: Memories from bygone era. Heart, Lung and Circulation. 2012;**21**(6–7):311-319

[10] Naser N. On occasion of seventy-five years of cardiac defibrillation in humans. Acta Inform Med. 2023;**31**(1):68-72

[11] Beaudouin D, Kouwenhoven WB. Reviving the Body Electric. JHU Engineering. Fall; 2022

[12] Wikipedia. Claude Beck. Available from: https://en.wikipedia.org/wiki/Claude_Beck

[13] Cohen SI. Paul M. Zoll, MD - the father of "modern" electrotherapy and innovator of pharmacotherapy for life-threatening cardiac arrhythmias. Resuscitation. 2007;**73**(2):178-185

[14] Lown B. Available from: https://lowninstitute.org/about/dr-bernard-lown/

[15] Cadogan M. Frank Pantridge. Life in Fastline. 03.11.2020. Available from: https://litfl.com/frank-pantridge/

[16] Kouwenhoven WB. The development of the defibrillator. Annals of Internal Medicine. 1969;**71**(3):449-458

[17] Eiggers CD. Diagram showing cardiac pressures, volume and electrical activity with corresponding phonocardiogram. Available from: https://www.researchgate.net/publication/338572639_CardioScope_ECG_sonification_and_auditory_augmentation_of_heart_sounds_to_support_cardiac_diagnostic_and_monitoring/figures?lo=1

[18] Wiggers CJ. The Physiological Society. 14/10/2019 Available from:

https://www.physoc.org/honorary_member/carl-j-wiggers/

[19] Wegria R, Wiggers CJ. Factors determining the production of ventricular fibrillation by direct currents. (with a note on chronaxie). American Heart Journal (Elsevier). 1940;**20**(4):399-412

[20] Cakulev I, Efimov IR, Waldo AL. Cardioversion: Past, present, and future. Circulation. 2009;**120**(16):1623-1632

[21] Diack AW, Welborn WS, Rullman RG, Walter CW, Wayne MA. An automatic cardiac resuscitator for emergency treatment of cardiac arrest. Medical Instrumentation. 1979;**13**(2): 78-83

[22] Bachman JW, McDonald GS, O'Brien PC. A study of out-of-hospital cardiac arrests in northeastern Minnesota. Journal of the American Medical Association. 1986;**256**(4): 477-483

[23] Cummins RO, Eisenberg MS, Litwin PE, Graves JR, Hearne TR, Hallstrom AP. Automatic external defibrillators used by emergency medical technicians. A controlled clinical trial. Journal of the American Medical Association. 1987;**257**(12):1605-1610

[24] Weaver WD, Hill D, Fahrenbruch CE, Copass MK, Martin JS, Cobb LA, et al. Use of the automatic external defibrillator in the management of out-of-hospital cardiac arrest. The New England Journal of Medicine. 1988;**319**(11):661-666

[25] Stults KR, Drown DD, Kerber RE. Efficacy of an automated external defibrillator in the management of out-of-hospital cardiac arrest: Validation of the diagnostic algorithm and initial clinical experience in a rural environment. Circulation. 1986;**73**(4): 701-709

[26] Vukov LF, White RD, Bachman JW, O'Brien PC. New perspectives on rural EMT defibrillation. Annals of Emergency Medicine. 1988;**17**(4): 318-321

[27] White SJ, Hamilton WA, Veronesi JF. A comparison of field techniques used to pressure-infuse intravenous fluids. Prehospital and Disaster Medicine. 1991;**6**(4):415-412

[28] Stapczynski JS, Svenson JE, Stone CK. Population density, automated external defibrillator use, and survival in rural cardiac arrest. Academic Emergency Medicine. 1997;**4**(6):552-558

[29] Whitney-Cashio P, Sartin M, Brady WJ, Williamson K, Alibertis K, Somers G, et al. The introduction of public access defibrillation to a university community: The University of Virginia public access defibrillation program. The American Journal of Emergency Medicine. 2012;**30**(6):e1-e8

[30] Valenzuela TD, Roe DJ, Nichol G, Clark LL, Spaite DW, Hardman RG. Outcomes of rapid defibrillation by security officers after cardiac arrest in casinos. The New England Journal of Medicine. 2000;**343**(17):1206-1209

[31] England H, Hoffman C, Hodgman T, Singh S, Homoud M, Weinstock J, et al. Effectiveness of automated external defibrillators in high schools in greater Boston. The American Journal of Cardiology. 2005;**95**(12):1484-1486

[32] Ruan Y, Sun G, Li C, An Y, Yue L, Zhu M, et al. Accessibility of automatic external defibrillators and survival rate of people with out-of-hospital cardiac arrest: A systematic review of real-world studies. Resuscitation. 2021;**167**:200-208

[33] Zuratynski P, Slezak D, Dabrowski S, Krzyzanowski K, Medrzycka-Dabrowska W, Rutkowski P. Use of public automated external defibrillators in out-of-hospital cardiac arrest in Poland. Medicina. 2021;**57**:298

[34] Schneider T, Martens PR, Paschen H. Multicenter, randomized, controlled trial of 150-J biphasic shocks compared with 200- to 360-J monophasic shocks in the resuscitation of out-of-hospital cardiac arrest victims. Circulation. 2000;**102**(15):1780-1787

[35] Greene HL, DiMarco JP, Kudenchuk PJ, Scheinman MM, Tang AS, Reiter MJ, et al. Comparison of monophasic and biphasic defibrillating pulse waveforms for transthoracic cardioversion. Biphasic waveform defibrillation investigators. The American Journal of Cardiology. 1995; **75**(16):1135-1139

[36] Weaver WD, Martin JS, Wirkus MJ, Morud S, Vincent S, Litwin PE, et al. Influence of external defibrillator electrode polarity on cardiac resuscitation. Pacing and Clinical Electrophysiology. 1993;**16**(2):285-290

[37] Available from: https://www.accessdata.fda.gov/scripts/cdrh/cfdocs/cfpma/pma.cfm?id=P160008

Section 2

Electrical and Drug Therapy of Arrhythmogenic Heart Diseases

Chapter 3

ICD for Sudden Cardiac Death Prevention and New Pharmaceutical Treatment Options in Hypertrophic Obstructive Cardiomyopathy

Antonio da Silva Menezes Junior, Thais Aratak Marques Taia, Camila Cássia Canzi, Ana Lígia Valeriano de Oliveira, Lucas Eduardo Almeida França, Aline Lins da Silva, Matheus Araújo Borges and Guilherme Diniz Prudente

Abstract

In humans, hypertrophic cardiomyopathy (HCM) is a heterogeneous cardiac illness typically caused by autosomal dominant sarcomeric gene mutations and characterized by reduced heart's compliance, myofibrillar disarray, and fibrosis of the heart. Areas covered: Although HCM was formerly viewed as a malignant disease entity with few treatment choices, effective management strategies have emerged so that affected individuals may expect to have a normal lifespan without the need for pacing or another type of invasive intervention. Herein, these management strategies are discussed. There is no curative treatment for HCM that reverses or prevents hypertrophy and heart dysfunction. Drug-based therapies aim to alleviate its symptoms and slow disease progression. Mavacamten is a reversible cardiac myosin allosteric modulator with a potential therapeutic effect for obstructive HCM. Mavacamten markedly improved the health status of patients with symptomatic obstructive hypertrophic cardiomyopathy compared with a placebo. In patients with HOCM, the importance of an implantable cardioverter defibrillators (ICD) is to prevent sudden cardiac death (SCD). Approximately 25% of those with HCM suffer from atrial arrhythmias, and the condition is notoriously difficult to manage. Anti-arrhythmic drugs, such as sotalol, amiodarone, and disopyramide, are routinely prescribed. Radiofrequency ablations for atrial fibrillation in patients with HCM have become more common despite their limited effectiveness (about 70% recurrence).

Keywords: obstructive hypertrophic cardiomyopathy, implantable cardioverter Desfibrillator, sudden cardiac death, pharmaceutical treatment, prevention

1. Introduction

In humans, hypertrophic cardiomyopathy (HCM) is a common (1:500 – general population) autosomal dominant inherited cardiovascular disease. It is caused by more than 1400 mutations in 11 or more genes encoding proteins of the cardiac sarcomere. HCM is characterized by left ventricular (LV) hypertrophy, myocardial hypercontractility, and other cardiac abnormalities. Reduced compliance, myofibrillar disarray, and fibrosis are all fenotypes of HCM [1, 2].

Even though HCM was formerly seen as a bleak, unyielding, and malignant disease entity with few treatment choices, the clinical story of the illness has dramatically transformed in recent years. Improved clinical recognition, including benign low-risk subgroups without significant symptoms or disability [3] has led to effective management strategies for major HCM complications, resulting in significantly lower mortality and morbidity rates. Affected individuals have an increased likelihood of achieving normal longevity into their 70s to 90s or even later with good quality of life [3].

Patients with LV dysfunction, obstruction of the left ventricular outflow tract (LVOT), and mitral regurgitation (MR) may have impaired exercise capacity, as well as exertional dyspnea and chest discomfort and syncope. Microvascular dysfunction and subendocardial ischemia are the underlying causes of these symptoms. Septal hypertrophy, as well as issues with the mitral valve and subvalvular apparatus, contribute to systolic anterior motion (SAM) and obstruction of the LVOT, resulting in obstructive HCM (HOCM), as seen in **Table 1**.

2. Implantable defibrillator cardioverter

Implantable cardioverter defibrillators (ICDs), composed of a defibrillator and electrodes, avoid ventricular arrhythmias and sudden death. The American Heart Association (AHA) and the European Society of Cardiology (ESC) recommend ICDs as a secondary preventive measure for patients with hemodynamically severe ventricular arrhythmias or prior cardiac arrests, as seen in **Table 2** and **Figure 1** [4].

Studies demonstrate that an ICD helps individuals who have had cardiac arrests and slows the progression of HCM by averting sudden death [1, 2]. In patients with HOCM, biventricular implanted cardio defibrillators reduce obstruction in the LVOT, indicating that they improve systolic function in the left ventricle [5].

Thavikulwat et al. studied adult patients with HCM treated with ICD at the Cardiovascular Institute of Bluhm from 2000 to 2013 to assess risk factor profiles, ICD treatment rates, and consequences [4]. During the 5.2-year period, 25 of the 135 patients treated received ICDs. No statistically significant difference was observed between individuals who died suddenly and those who did not undergo ICD therapy. While younger ICD patients received more suitable care, 20% of these patients had insufficient therapy.

Maron et al. [5] studied 486 individuals with high-risk HCM from eight worldwide sites. Among them, 19% received ICD intervention due to ventricular tachycardia or fibrillation. Only one patient died suddenly from ICD failure, while three others died from causes connected to HCM but unrelated to the arrhythmogenic effect. Although anticipation of future shocks increased anxiety, individuals who received any ICD intervention showed no HCM mortality in 1, 5, and 10 years [5]. Notably, ICD was not associated with an increase in mortality, cardiovascular

Structural Derangements	Molecular Derangements	Novel Procedures	Novel Pharmacotherapies	Gene-Based Therapies	Genetic Derangements
Septal hypertrophy	Actin-myosin cross-bridging	Surgical papillary muscle realignment, chordae removal, and mitral valve repair	Mavacamten, CK-274	Allele-specific gene silencing	Genetic mutations in sarcomeric proteins
Mitral leaflet abnormalities	Myocardial metabolism Sodium and calcium channels	Apical myectomy	Perhexiline, trimetazidine ranolazine, eleclazine N-acetylcysteine ARBs, aldosterone antagonists	Embryonic gene repair using CRISPR/Cas9	—
Subvalvular abnormalities	Hyperdynamic L function, impaired LV relaxation and compliance	Transcatheter mitral valve repair	Statins	—	—
SAM/LOT obstruction	Myocardial disarray, fibrosis, and adverse remodeling	Radiofrequency septal ablation	—	—	—
Mitral regurgitation	—	High-intensity focused ultrasound septal ablation	—	—	—

Novel procedural approaches target cardiac structural abnormalities in hypertrophic cardiomyopathy. Novel pharmacotherapies target abnormal cellular processes in hypertrophic cardiomyopathy. Allele-specific gene silencing and genome editing using CRISPR/Cas9 target the genetic underpinnings of hypertrophic cardiomyopathy. ARB, angiotensin II receptor blocker; LV, left ventricular; LVOT, left ventricular outflow tract; SAM, systolic anterior motion. Source: Tuohy CV, Kaul S, Song HK, Nazer B, Heitner SB. Hypertrophic cardiomyopathy: the future of treatment. Eur J Heart Fail. 2020;22(2):228–240. doi:10.1002/ejhf.1715 Order Date12-May-2022/Order License ID1220726–1/ISSN1388–9842.

Table 1.
Novel therapeutic targets in hypertrophic cardiomyopathy.

Class of recommendation	Recommendations
1 – Strong	In patients with HCM, individualization is recommended, with prognostic analysis of conventional risk markers, clinical profile, and balanced discussion of evidence, risks, and benefits, involving the patient actively in the decision-making process for implantation of the ICD.
1 – Strong	ICD implantation is recommended in patients with HCM and a history of documented cardiac arrest or sustained ventricular tachycardia (VT)
2ª – Moderate	It is reasonable to offer an ICD implant to adult patients with HCM with ≥1 major risk factor, as listed below, for sudden cardiac death. a. Sudden cardiac death judged definitive or likely attributed to HCM in ≥1 first-degree relatives or close relatives aged ≤50 years. b. Massive LVH ≥30 mm in any left ventricular (LV) segment; c. Presence of ≥1 suspicious episode of syncope, such that its origin is neurocardiogenic (vasovagal) or related to Left ventricular outflow tract obstruction (LVOTO); d. LV apical aneurysm, independent of size; e. LV systolic dysfunction (EF <50%).
2ª – Moderate	ICD implantation becomes reasonable in children with HCM with ≥1 conventional risk factor, including unexplained syncope, massive LVH, NSTV, or family history of HCM related to early sudden cardiac death (SCD);
2ª – Moderate	For patients≥16 years of age with HCM and with ≥1 major SCD risk factor, discussion of the estimated 5-year risk of sudden cardiac death and mortality rates may prove helpful during the shared decision-making process for placement of the CDI
2b – Weak	Selected adult patients who have HCM and do not have risk factors for sudden cardiac death after clinical evaluation, or in whom the decision to proceed with ICD implantation still remains uncertain, ICD can be considered in patients with extensive Late Gadolinium Enhancement (LGE) by cardiac magnetic resonance (CMR) or nonsustained ventricular tachycardia (NSTV) present on ambulatory monitoring
2b – Weak	For selected pediatric patients with HCM and uncertain risk stratification, it may be worth considering additional factors such as extensive Late Gadolinium Enhancement (LGE) on cardiovascular magnetic resonance imaging (CMR) and systolic dysfunction in risk stratification
3 – Harm	ICD placement should not be performed in patients with HCM without risk factors
3 – Harm	In patients with HCM, ICD placement for the sole purpose of participation in competitive athletics should not be performed

The original source was adapted from the authors. "Ommen SR, Mital S, Burke MA, Day SM, Deswal A, Elliott P, et al. 2020 AHA/ACC Guideline for the Diagnosis and Treatment of Patients with Hypertrophic Cardiomyopathy: Executive Summary: A Report of the American College of Cardiology/American Heart Association Joint Committee on Clinical Practice Guidelines. Vol. 142, Circulation. Lippincott Williams and Wilkins; 2020. p. E533–57."

Table 2.
Eligibility criteria for ICD implementation.

morbidity, or worsening heart failure. Furthermore, although it causes worry in people who have previously received ICD intervention, it does not significantly affect their psychological well-being [5].

Giraldeau et al., despite studying a small sample, assessed the effectiveness of biventricular stimulation (BiV) in 13 individuals (average age of 55 years) with

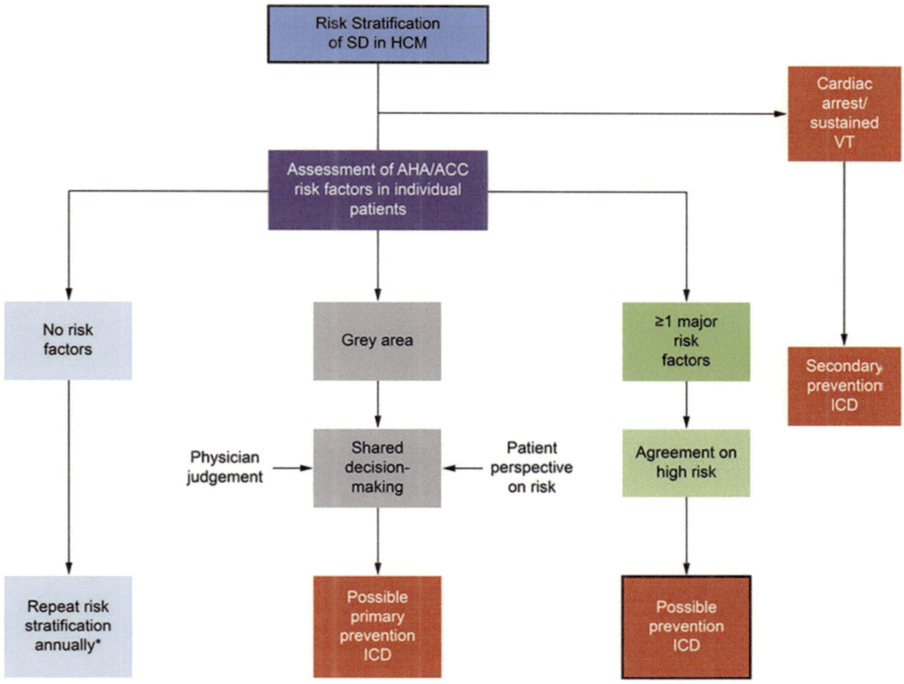

Figure 1.
Risk stratification of SD in HCM. HCM = hypertrophic cardiomyopathy; ICD = implantable cardioverter defibrillator; SD = sudden death; VT = ventricular tachycardia. Source: Maron BJ, Desai MY, Nishimura RA, et al. Management of Hypertrophic Cardiomyopathy: JACC state-of-the-art review. J Am Coll Cardiol. 2022; 79:390–414. This agreement between Antonio da Silva Menezes junior ("You") and Elsevier ("Elsevier") consists of your license details and the terms and conditions provided by Elsevier and copyright clearance center. License number 5305400128072 license date may 10, 2022.

HOCM who had undergone 2D transthoracic echocardiography before implantation and were followed for 12 months [6]. The peak gradient in the LVOT was lowered from 80 to 30 mmHg. Displacement curve analysis revealed an inversion of lateral wall movement time in these individuals, with a reduced LVOT gradient. The study concluded that BiV reduces LVL obstruction in patients with HOCM by desynchronizing LV movement and inverting the activation time of the LV wall, without affecting the LV's systolic function [6].

To diagnose, confirm, or stratify the type of hypertrophy present in individuals with HCM, Freitas et al. conducted a multicentric retrospective investigation of 493 patients (58% male; mean age of 46 years) [7]. Their goal was to prove that cardiovascular magnetic resonance imaging and late gadolinium enhancement may be used to stratify risk. The sudden death risk score for HCM and the algorithms of the American College of Cardiology Foundation and the American Association of Cardiology (ACCF/AHA) were used to determine individuals' eligibility for ICDs. During the median 3.4-year follow-up, 12 patients died, 6 had adequate ICD discharges, and 5 had prolonged ventricular tachycardia. Compared to ratings and algorithms, late gadolinium enhancement was the sole independent predictor of outcomes. As people with HCM are more prone to unexpected death, this tool is vital.

Aducci et al. [8] studied 77 patients (45 male, mean age of 46 years) with HCM who received a transvenous ICD. In total, 24 of the patients experienced 49 episodes

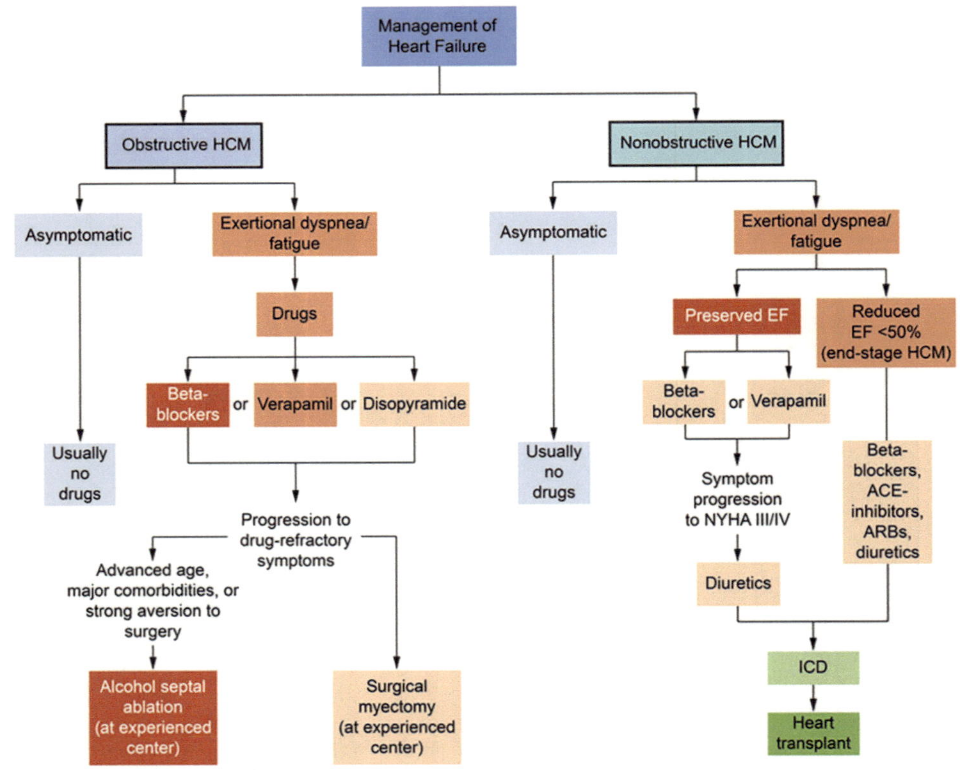

Figure 2.
Management strategies for HCM. HCM = hypertrophic cardiomyopathy; ICD = implantable cardioverter defibrillator; SD = sudden death; VT = ventricular tachycardia. Source: Maron BJ, Desai MY, Nishimura RA, et al. Management of Hypertrophic Cardiomyopathy: JACC state-of-the-art review. J Am Coll Cardiol. 2022; 79:390–414. This agreement between Antonio da Silva Menezes junior ("You") and Elsevier ("Elsevier") consists of your license details and the terms and conditions provided by Elsevier and copyright clearance center. License number 5305400128072 license date may 10, 2022.

of ventricular tachycardia/fibrillation after 67 months. Antitachycardia pacing (ATP) by ICD was successful in 69% of 39 monomorphic ventricular tachycardia (VT) events. However, even with ATP, two episodes of VT occurred. [8]. Thus, although ATP is relatively successful in treating monomorphic VTs in patients with HCM, its optimal treatment rate remains low, and it is typically provided prematurely, raising concerns about arrhythmia induced by ATP [8].

Between June 2014 and May 2016, Maurizi et al. [9] studied 50 patients (34 males; mean age of 40 years; body mass index [BMI] of 25.2) with HCM referred for subcutaneous ICD implantation in primary and secondary preventive centers in seven Italian locations. VT occurred in seven individuals and was cardioverted in two cases. The remaining patients experienced 73 bouts of ventricular fibrillation, with 6% spontaneous conversion. Defibrillation failed in only one patient, who was significantly obese (BMI of 36) and had a maximal LV wall thickness of 25 mm [9].

As reported by the AHA, the 65 J acute defibrillation test with subcutaneous ICD detects and stops VT in 98% of people. Severe obesity is the cause of lone failure (9). These recommendations and/or the ESC's HCM sudden cardiac death (SCD) risk calculator is used to determine if an ICD should be used in a patient at risk for SCD. Late gadolinium enhancement on cardiac magnetic resonance imaging, LV systolic dysfunction, and LV apical aneurysm have all been included in an American College of Cardiology (ACC)/AHA risk stratification strategy that has recently shown improved discrimination for SCD or appropriate ICD therapies, as seen in **Figure 2**. However, this much more conservative approach would lead to significantly higher ICD utilization [10–17].

From January 2005 to September 2016, Valzania et al. studied 99 patients (mean age of 53 years) with HCM who received an ICD at Karolinska University Hospital. In follow-up, 12 died from heart failure (HF), 6 from SCD, and 6 from other causes; 20% of the patients demonstrated occlusion of the LVOT due to HOCM, and primary prevention was the top indication for an ICD [10–12].

Apart from septal reduction treatment, people with HCM may expect to have a normal lifespan without the need for pacing, which is indicated only when LVOTO is present. As a result, the subcutaneous implantable cardioverter defibrillator (S-ICD; Boston Scientific, Minneapolis, MN, USA) has become a viable option for both primary and secondary prevention of SCD. Due to the sensing mechanism of the S-ICD's three subcutaneous vectors, QRS and T-wave anomalies in young patients pose constraints—prescreening failure rates for patients with HCM range from 14–38% due to T-waver sensing. However, shocks might still be inappropriate in 8–24% of patients even after proper screening; inappropriate shocks can occur due to factors such as the need for reprogramming and muscle noise due to myopotentials [18]. Therefore, cautious patient selection is required [9, 10].

In patients with HOCM, the importance of an ICD is to avoid SCD (DDD ICD with a lead placed into RVA and programmed short AV-delay). Approximately 25% of those with HCM suffer from atrial arrhythmias, and the condition is notoriously difficult to manage. Anti-arrhythmic drugs, such as sotalol, amiodarone, and disopyramide, are routinely prescribed. Radiofrequency ablations for atrial fibrillation in patients with HCM have become more common despite their limited effectiveness (about 70% recurrence over 3–4 years after a single treatment). Myectomy surgery may be somewhat more successful than surgical ablation at the time of the procedure (recurrence rate of 36–51%), as seen in **Figure 2** [10–13].

3. Novel drugs for HCM

There is no curative treatment for HCM that reverses or prevents hypertrophy and heart dysfunction, but there are therapeutic options that can generate less progression and greater relief of symptoms. Therefore, drug-based therapies are aimed at alleviating the symptoms associated with HCM and slowing disease progression. Patients with HCM who are symptomatic are generally offered first-line pharmacotherapy with β-blockers or nondihydropyridine calcium channel blockers. Disopyramide is effective as an add-on therapy, although it can be poorly tolerated. The inotropic effects of these drugs have been the cornerstone of therapy for decades, reducing SAM/septal contact and LVOT occlusion. However, existing guideline-directed pharmacotherapies were never developed for the treatment of HCM, and lack of evidence. Further, randomized studies have not shown the superiority of any treatment over that of the placebo, based on a small study performed in 1966 [13]. Nonobstructive HCM (noHCM), which accounts for about 30% of all cases of HCM, remains poorly understood and has no recognized disease-modifying therapy. Studies have shown significant disparities in the presentation of HCM between men and women, with the latter being older and more symptomatic at the time of diagnosis, as well as perhaps having a poorer overall survival rate than the former [14–36].

3.1 Mavacantem and Aficatem (CK-274)

Mavacantem is a reversible cardiac myosin allosteric modulator that has a potential therapeutic effect for individuals with (HOCM). This modulator demonstrated significant mitigation of hypercontractility, ventricular hypertrophy, myofibrillar disarrangement, and fibrosis in animal models [36–43].

Patients with HCM were treated with mavacamten for 12 weeks, which resulted in a quick and significant decrease in the gradient (LVOT) following exercise in the study participants. Patients with plasma mavacamten concentrations between 350 ng/mL and 700 ng/mL were more likely to have a VSVE gradient of less than 30 mmHg (the threshold for obstruction in HCM) and less than 50 mmHg (the threshold for consideration of septal reduction therapy) than those with lower values. Such an event is probably due to the fact that mavacamten acts to reduce the formation of actin-myosin cross-bridges, thus generating less systolic and diastolic cross-bridge formation. In addition, it promotes a relaxed energy-saving state that reduces LVOT obstruction [21]. A clinically significant improvement in symptoms, particularly dyspnea, as well as increased effort capacity, was also observed [44, 45]. At the end of the 12-week research, mavacamten lowered the mean gradient of postexercise VSVE from 103 mmHg (standard deviation, 50) at baseline to 19 mmHg (standard deviation, 13; mean change, −89.5 mmHg; 95% confidence interval [CI], −138.3 to - 40.7 mm Hg; P = 0.008). The LVEF at rest was also decreased (mean variation, −15%; CI, −23% to −6%), while peak oxygen consumption rose by an average of 3.5 mL/kg/min (CI 1.2 to 5.9 mL/kg/min) [44–46].

While this modulator was well tolerated by patients at exposures that successfully decreased VSVE obstruction, decreases in LVEF that were greater than those required to alleviate VESV obstruction were shown to be irreversible. Lowered LVEF at higher plasma concentrations and atrial fibrillation (AF) were the most prevalent adverse events conclusively or probably associated with mavacamten use [46].

Several characteristics of HCM were demonstrated by Prondzynski et al. [47], including hypertrophy, myofibrillar disarray, hypercontractility, impaired relaxation, and increased myofilament mass. They also demonstrated that cardiomyocytes derived from human induced pluripotent stem cells and manipulated cardiac tissues recapitulated several characteristics of HCM, including prolongation of the duration of the action potential and increase in myofilament, among others. As a result of these differences, the current density of calcium channel type L was greater in those with HCM than in the control group, as was the duration of the action potential. In addition to the above, this study revealed a novel HCM mutation that was associated with a contractile and electrophysiological phenotype in hiPSC-derived cardiomyocytes [47–57].

It was revealed via the optimization of the indoline compound that aficamten (CK-274), a new cardiac myosin inhibitor, could be developed. Among the most significant advancements in the optimization process was the identification of an Indane analog, which is a molecule that presents an attractive biological profile for the development of therapeutic molecules, in such a way that having a less restricted structure-activity relationship and allowing the fast development of drug-like characteristics. Aficamten was developed to have a predicted human half-life (t1/2) appropriate for once daily (od) dosing, to reach a steady state in less than two weeks, to cause no significant cytochrome P450 induction or inhibition, and to have a broad therapeutic window in vivo with a clear pharmacokinetic/pharmacodynamic relationship, among other characteristics. Aficamten displayed a human t1/2 that was comparable to projections in the phase I clinical study, and it was able to achieve steady state concentration within the two-week timeframe that had been set [58].

With an estimated human half-life of two weeks and no significant CYP induction or inhibition in preclinical studies, aficamten offers an attractive therapeutic window and a clear PK/PD connection. The large therapeutic window reported in preclinical trials seems to apply to people, supporting the development of aficamten into phase 1 investigations. Aficamten may help reduce cardiac sarcomere hypercontractility, which seems to cause pathological hypertrophy, outflow obstruction, and fibrosis in some hereditary hypertrophic cardiomyopathies [18, 58, 59].

4. Conclusions

There is no curative treatment for HCM that reverses or prevents hypertrophy and heart dysfunction; therefore, drug-based therapies are aimed at alleviating the symptoms associated with HCM and slowing disease progression. Notably, ICD is beneficial for the prevention of SCD, as it is not associated with an increase in mortality, cardiovascular morbidity, or worsening of HF. While people who have previously experienced some type of ICD intervention express anxiety, it does not significantly affect their psychological well-being.

In certain cases, implanting ICDs is a difficult choice to make, particularly when the available information is insufficient to appropriately classify a patient's risk level. To resolve the doubt, a thorough physician's clinical judgment/intuition and medical reasoning, as well as frank discussions with fully informed patients and families, considering the benefits and limitations of risk stratification and ICDs, may be beneficial. In this approach, the different personal views of patients about sudden death risk and implanted gadgets, as well as opinions from other countries and cultures, are to be considered. The risk of sudden death in HCM is the same for men and women of any race or gender, although ICDs are less often used in minorities than in majority populations.

A successful treatment/prevention of life-threatening ventricular arrhythmias in the HCM population has been proven despite the severe morphology typical of HCM, which often includes large degrees of left ventricular hypertrophy and/or LV outflow tract obstruction. A high incidence of appropriate intervention was seen in studies of individuals judged to be at high risk, both in secondary prevention and in primary prevention, the researchers found. It is even more remarkable that this adequate intervention rate is achieved even considering the young and generally healthy individuals that make up the HCM population.

Because the incidence of SCD in HCM is very low, it is critical to identify individuals who are at high risk of SCD. Traditional risk classification strategies based on clinical risk variables have significant drawbacks and have been shown to overestimate the level of risk. Compared to standard risk prediction models based on bivariate risk variables, a novel risk prediction model that delivers individual 5-year projected risk seems to be better. Preoperative problems seem to be comparable to those associated with the placement of other cardiac devices, but long-term consequences have typically been the focus of research and discussion. Because of their young age at implant and higher frequency of atrial fibrillation, HCM patients are assumed to be more prone to ICD-related issues and inappropriate ICD treatment. However, long-term follow-up evidence on ICD-related complications in general practice is sparse.

Conflict of interest

The authors declare no conflict of interest.

Author details

Antonio da Silva Menezes Junior*, Thais Aratak Marques Taia, Camila Cássia Canzi, Ana Lígia Valeriano de Oliveira, Lucas Eduardo Almeida França, Aline Lins da Silva, Matheus Araújo Borges and Guilherme Diniz Prudente
Medical and Life School Goiânia, Pontifical Catholic University of Goiás, Goiás, Brazil

*Address all correspondence to: a.menezes.junior@uol.com.br

IntechOpen

© 2023 The Author(s). Licensee IntechOpen. This chapter is distributed under the terms of the Creative Commons Attribution License (http://creativecommons.org/licenses/by/3.0), which permits unrestricted use, distribution, and reproduction in any medium, provided the original work is properly cited.

References

[1] Maron BJ. Clinical course and management of hypertrophic cardiomyopathy. The New England Journal of Medicine. 2018;**379**:655-668

[2] Spudich JA. Three perspectives on the molecular basis of hypercontractility caused by hypertrophic cardiomyopathy mutations. Pflügers Archiv. 2019;**471**:701-717

[3] Maron BJ, Desai MY, Nishimura RA, et al. Management of hypertrophic cardiomyopathy: JACC state-of-the-art review. Journal of the American College of Cardiology. 2022;**79**:390-414

[4] Thavikulwat AC, Tomson TT, Knight BP, et al. Appropriate implantable defibrillator therapy in adults with hypertrophic cardiomyopathy. Journal of Cardiovascular Electrophysiology. 2016;**27**:953-960

[5] Maron BJ, Casey SA, Olivotto I, et al. Clinical course and quality of life in high-risk patients with hypertrophic cardiomyopathy and implantable cardioverter-defibrillators, 2018, 11(4):e005820. Circulation. Arrhythmia and Electrophysiology DOI: 10.1161/CIRCEP.117.005820. 2018;11:1-9

[6] Sanchez DJ, Lozano IF. Implantable cardioverter-defibrillator in hypertrophic cardiomyopathy. Global Cardiology Science & Practice. 2018;**31**:1-22. DOI: 10.21542/GCSP.2018.31

[7] Giraldeau G, Duchateau N, Bijnens B, et al. Dyssynchronization reduces dynamic obstruction without affecting systolic function in patients with hypertrophic obstructive cardiomyopathy: A pilot study. The International Journal of Cardiovascular Imaging. 2016;**32**:1179-1188

[8] Freitas P, Ferreira AM, Arteaga-Fernández E, et al. The amount of late gadolinium enhancement outperforms current guideline-recommended criteria in the identification of patients with hypertrophic cardiomyopathy at risk of sudden cardiac death. Journal of Cardiovascular Magnetic Resonance. 2019;**21**:50-60. DOI: 10.1186/s12968-019-0561-4

[9] Adduci C, Semprini L, Palano F, et al. Safety and efficacy of anti-tachycardia pacing in patients with hypertrophic cardiomyopathy implanted with an ICD. Pacing and Clinical Electrophysiology. 2019;**42**:610-616

[10] Maurizi N et al. Effectiveness of subcutaneous implantable cardioverter-defibrillator testing in patients with hypertrophic cardiomyopathy. International Journal of Cardiology. 2017;**31**:115-119

[11] Valzania C et al. Cardiac implantable electrical devices in patients with hypertrophic cardiomyopathy: Single center implant data extracted from the Swedish pacemaker and ICD registry. Scandinavian Cardiovascular Journal. 2020;**54**:239-247

[12] Tuohy CV, Kaul S, Song HK, et al. Hypertrophic cardiomyopathy: The future of treatment. European Journal of Heart Failure. 2020;**22**:228-240

[13] Atkuri KR, Mantovani JJ, Herzenberg LA, et al. N-acetylcysteine–a safe antidote for cysteine/glutathione deficiency. Current Opinion in Pharmacology. 2007;**7**:355-359

[14] Lombardi R, Rodriguez G, Chen SN, et al. Resolution of established cardiac

hypertrophy and fibrosis and prevention of systolic dysfunction in a transgenic rabbit model of human cardiomyopathy through thiol-sensitive mechanisms. Circulation. 2009;**119**:1398-1407

[15] Senthil V, Chen SN, Tsybouleva N, et al. Prevention of cardiac hypertrophy by atorvastatin in a transgenic rabbit model of human hypertrophic cardiomyopathy. Circulation Research. 2005;**97**:285-292

[16] Takimoto E, Kass DA. Role of oxidative stress in cardiac hypertrophy and remodeling. Hypertension. 2007;**49**:241-248

[17] Marian AJ, Senthil V, Chen SN, et al. Antifibrotic effects of antioxidant N-acetylcysteine in a mouse model of human hypertrophic cardiomyopathy mutation. Journal of the American College of Cardiology. 2006;**47**:827-834

[18] Maria E, Olaru A, Cappelli S. The entirely subcutaneous defibrillator (S-Icd): State of the art and selection of the ideal candidate. Current Cardiology Reviews. 2014;**11**:180-186

[19] Horowitz JD, Chirkov YY. Perhexiline and hypertrophic cardiomyopathy: A new horizon for metabolic modulation. Circulation. 2010;**122**:1547-1549

[20] Kennedy JA, Unger SA, Horowitz JD. Inhibition of carnitine palmitoyltransferase-1 in rat heart and liver by perhexiline and amiodarone. Biochemical Pharmacology. 1996;**52**:273-280

[21] Anderson RL, Trivedi DV, Sarkar SS, Henze M, Ma W, Gong H, et al. Deciphering the super relaxed state of human β-cardiac myosin and the mode of action of mavacamten from myosin molecules to muscle fibers. Proceedings of the National Academy of Sciences of the United States of America. 2018;**115**:8143-8152

[22] Ashrafian H, McKenna WJ, Watkins H. Disease pathways and novel therapeutic targets in hypertrophic cardiomyopathy. Circulation Research. 2011;**109**:86-96

[23] Ashrafian H, Redwood C, Blair E, et al. Hypertrophic cardiomyopathy: A paradigm for myocardial energy depletion. Trends in Genetics. 2003;**19**:263-268

[24] Olivotto I, Hellawell JL, Farzaneh-Far R, et al. Novel approach targeting the complex pathophysiology of hypertrophic cardiomyopathy: The impact of late sodium current inhibition on exercise capacity in subjects with symptomatic hypertrophic cardiomyopathy (LIBERTY-HCM) trial. Circulation. Heart Failure. 2016;**9**:1-10

[25] Abozguia K, Elliott P, McKenna W, et al. Metabolic modulator perhexiline corrects energy deficiency and improves exercise capacity in symptomatic hypertrophic cardiomyopathy. Circulation. 2010;**122**:1562-1569

[26] Ananthakrishna R et al. Randomized controlled trial of perhexiline on regression of left ventricular hypertrophy in patients with symptomatic hypertrophic cardiomyopathy (RESOLVE-HCM trial). American Heart Journal. 2021;**240**:101-113

[27] Warshaw DM. Throttling back the heart's molecular motor. A small molecule inhibits mutated forms of myosin that cause cardiac hypertrophy. Science. 2016;**351**:556-557

[28] Green EM, Wakimoto H, Anderson RL, et al. A small-molecule inhibitor of sarcomere contractility suppresses hypertrophic cardiomyopathy in mice. Science. 2016;**351**:617-621

[29] Andries G, Yandrapalli S, Naidu SS, et al. Novel pharmacotherapy in hypertrophic cardiomyopathy. Cardiology in Review. 2018;**26**:239-244

[30] Authors/Task Force Members, Elliott PM, Anastasakis A, et al. ESC guidelines on diagnosis and management of hypertrophic cardiomyopathy: The task force for the diagnosis and management of hypertrophic cardiomyopathy of the European Society of Cardiology (ESC). European Heart Journal. 2014;**2014**(35):2733-2779

[31] Spoladore R, Maron MS, D'Amato R, et al. Pharmacological treatment options for hypertrophic cardiomyopathy: High time for evidence. European Heart Journal. 2012;**33**:1724-1733

[32] Tsybouleva N, Zhang L, Chen S, et al. Aldosterone, through novel signaling proteins, is a fundamental molecular bridge between the genetic defect and the cardiac phenotype of hypertrophic cardiomyopathy. Circulation. 2004;**109**:1284-1291

[33] Orenes-Piñero E, Hernández-Romero D, Jover E, et al. Impact of polymorphisms in the renin-angiotensin-aldosterone system on hypertrophic cardiomyopathy. Journal of the Renin-Angiotensin-Aldosterone System. 2011;**12**:521-530

[34] De Resende MM, Kriegel AJ, Greene AS. Combined effects of low-dose spironolactone and captopril therapy in a rat model of genetic hypertrophic cardiomyopathy. Journal of Cardiovascular Pharmacology. 2006;**48**:265-273

[35] Kawano H, Toda G, Nakamizo R, et al. Valsartan decreases typeI collagen synthesis in patients with hypertrophic cardiomyopathy. Circulation Journal. 2005;**69**:1244-1248

[36] Araujo AQ, Arteaga E, Ianni BM, et al. Effect of losartan on left ventricular diastolic function in patients with nonobstructive hypertrophic cardiomyopathy. The American Journal of Cardiology. 2005;**96**:1563-1567

[37] Yamazaki T, Suzuki J, Shimamoto RA, et al. A new therapeutic strategy for hypertrophic nonobstructive cardiomyopathy in humans. A randomized and prospective study with an angiotensin II receptor blocker. International Heart Journal. 2007;**48**:715-724

[38] Penicka M, Gregor P, Kerekes R, et al. The effects of candesartan on left ventricular hypertrophy and function in nonobstructive hypertrophic cardiomyopathy: A pilot, randomized study. The Journal of Molecular Diagnostics. 2009;**11**:35-41

[39] Maltês S, Lopes LR. New perspectives in the pharmacological treatment of hypertrophic cardiomyopathy. Revista Portuguesa de Cardiologia (English edition). 2020;**39**:99-109

[40] Coppini R, Ferrantini C, Yao L, et al. Late sodium current inhibition reverses electromechanical dysfunction in human hypertrophic cardiomyopathy. Circulation. 2013;**127**:575-584

[41] Olivotto I, Camici PG, Merlini PA, et al. Efficacy of ranolazine in patients with symptomatic hypertrophic cardiomyopathy: The RESTYLE-HCM randomized, double-blind, placebo-controlled study. Circulation. Heart Failure. 2018;**11**:1-10

[42] Kostner KM. Statin therapy for hypertrophic cardiomyopathy: Too good to be true? European Journal of Clinical Investigation. 2010;**40**:965-967

[43] Liao JK, Laufs U. Pleiotropic effects of statins. Annual Review

of Pharmacology and Toxicology. 2005;**45**:89-118

[44] Simko F. Statins: A perspective for left ventricular hypertrophy treatment. European Journal of Clinical Investigation. 2007;**37**:681-691

[45] Nagueh SF, Lombardi R, Tan Y, et al. Atorvastatin and cardiac hypertrophy and function in hypertrophic cardiomyopathy: A pilot study. European Journal of Clinical Investigation. 2010;**40**:976-983

[46] Bauersachs J, Störk S, Kung M, et al. HMG CoA reductase inhibition and left ventricular mass in hypertrophic cardiomyopathy: A randomized placebo-controlled pilot study. European Journal of Clinical Investigation. 2007;**37**:852-859

[47] Prondzynski M, Lemoine MD, Zech AT, et al. Disease modeling of a mutation in α-actinin 2 guides clinical therapy in hypertrophic cardiomyopathy. EMBO Molecular Medicine. 2019;**11**:1-18

[48] Zampieri M, Berteotti M, Ferrantini C, et al. Pathophysiology and treatment of hypertrophic cardiomyopathy: New perspectives. Current Heart Failure Reports. 2021;**18**:169-179

[49] Li J, Wu Z, Zheng D, Sun Y, et al. Bioinformatics analysis of the regulatory lncRNA-miRNA-mRNA network and drug prediction in patients with hypertrophic cardiomyopathy. Molecular Medicine Reports. 2019;**20**:549-558

[50] Salman OF, El-Rayess HM, Abi Khalil C, Nemer G, Refaat MM. Inherited cardiomyopathies and the role of mutations in non-coding regions of the genome. Frontiers in Cardiovascular Medicine. 2018;**5**:1-12

[51] Kajimoto K, Otsubo S. Adding high-dose spironolactone to Tolvaptan improves acute decompensated heart failure due to obstructive hypertrophic cardiomyopathy and aortic stenosis: A case report. American Journal of Case Reports. 2019;**20**:1006-1010

[52] Tower-Rader A et al. Mavacamten: A novel small molecule modulator of β-cardiac myosin for treatment of hypertrophic cardiomyopathy. Expert Opinion on Investigational Drugs. 2020;**29**:1171-1178

[53] Olivotto I, Oreziak A, Barriales-Villa R, et al. Mavacamten for treatment of symptomatic obstructive hypertrophic cardiomyopathy (EXPLORER-HCM): A randomised, double-blind, placebo-controlled, phase 3 trial. Lancet (London, England). 2020;**2020**(396):759-769

[54] Imori Y, Takano H, Mase H, et al. Bisoprolol transdermal patch for perioperative care of non-cardiac surgery in patients with hypertrophic obstructive cardiomyopathy. BMC Cardiovascular Disorders. 2019;**19**:316-324

[55] Adler A, Fourey D, Weissler-Snir A, et al. Safety of outpatient initiation of disopyramide for obstructive hypertrophic cardiomyopathy patients. Journal of the American Heart Association. 2017;**6**:1-7

[56] de Oliveira GMM. A new look into hypertrophic cardiomyopathy based on clinical evidence. Revista Portuguesa de Cardiologia (English Edition). 2018;**37**:11-13

[57] Jung H, Yang PS, Jang E, et al. Effectiveness and safety of non-vitamin K antagonist oral anticoagulants in patients with atrial fibrillation with hypertrophic cardiomyopathy:

A nationwide cohort study. Chest. 2019;**155**:354-363

[58] Chuang C, Collibee S, Ashcraft L, Wang W, Vander Wal M, Wang X, et al. Discovery of Aficamten (CK-274), a next-generation cardiac myosin inhibitor for the treatment of hypertrophic cardiomyopathy. Journal of Medicinal Chemistry. 2021;**64**:14142-14152

[59] Heitner SB, Jacoby D, Lester SJ, et al. Mavacamten treatment for obstructive hypertrophic cardiomyopathy: A clinical trial. Annals of Internal Medicine. 2019;**170**:741-748

Chapter 4

Atrial Fibrillation and Cardioversion Drugs

Taomin Su, Pan Liu, Qin Shi, Yan Wang and Ying Zhou

Abstract

The heart is constantly and harmoniously alternating contractions and diastolic activities, and these mechanical activities are stimulated by the heart's electrical activity. Atrial fibrillation results in changes to atrial myocytes, with early but potentially reversible alteration in ion channels. Atrial fibrillation is one of the arrhythmias characterized by mechanical dysfunction caused by uncoordinated contraction of atrium, and it is also the most common and serious arrhythmia in clinical practice, which can cause serious complications, such as hemodynamic changes and cerebral embolism. Therefore, cardioversion drugs have become a research hotspot in the field of arrhythmia. Medical treatment of atrial fibrillation includes cardioversion, control of ventricular rate, and anticoagulation. This chapter focuses on drug cardioversion.

Keywords: atrial arrhythmias, atrial fibrillation, cardioversion drugs, heart, medical treatment

1. Introduction

The heart is constantly and harmoniously alternating contractions and diastolic activities, and these mechanical activities are stimulated by the heart's electrical activity. Atrial fibrillation results in changes to atrial myocytes, with early but potentially reversible alteration in ion channels. Later changes include structural remodeling with myocyte degeneration, myocardial fibrosis, left atrial enlargement, and heterogeneity of conduction [1]. The heart's electrical activity originates the sinus node, and the impulses are conducted to the right and left atrium, then to the atrioventricular node, and finally to the ventricular muscle along atrioventricular bundle, left and right bundle branches, and the Purkinje fiber network (shown in **Figure 1**). Cardiac arrhythmia occurs when the activity of the entire heart becomes too fast, too slow, or irregular or the sequence of activities of each part is disordered. Arrhythmias are classified in a wide variety of categories. According to its occurrence principle, it can be divided into two categories: abnormal impulse origin and abnormal impulse conduction. According to the site of origin, it can be divided into sinus, atrial, atrioventricular junction, and ventricular arrhythmia. According to the speed of heart rate during arrhythmia, it can be divided into fast and slow arrhythmia. Some scholars also propose to divide arrhythmias into two categories: benign and malignant, or lethal, potentially fatal and benign.

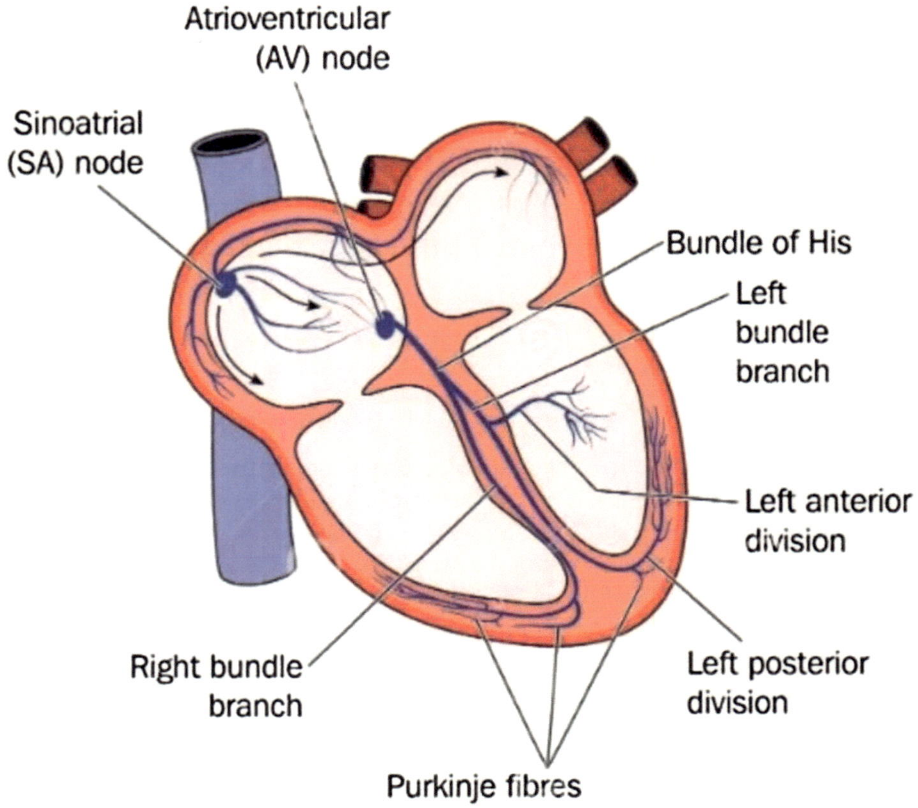

Figure 1.
Electrical activity of the heart.

2. Tachyarrhythmias

Tachyarrhythmias include premature atrial beats, atrial tachycardia (atrial tachycardia), atrial flutter (atrial flutter), and atrial fibrillation. Atrial fibrillation is the most common clinically significant arrhythmia, often associated with structural heart disease. Its prevalence increases with age and will continue to increase over the next 30 years, especially in countries with medium sociodemographic indices, becoming one of the greatest epidemic and public health challenges. Atrial fibrillation may cause hemodynamic disturbances and thromboembolic events. It has been reported that the prevalence of atrial fibrillation in the general population is 0.4 to 1.0%, the prevalence of people over 60 years old is 2–4%, and the incidence of elderly people over 80 years old can reach 8–10% [2]. When atrial fibrillation occurs, the auxiliary pump effect of the atria is lost, which reduces the cardiac output by 15–30%. This chapter mainly focuses on the pathogenesis of atrial fibrillation and its cardioversion drugs.

2.1 Epidemiology of atrial fibrillation

The number of cases of atrial fibrillation worldwide was estimated at 37.6 million in 2017 and is expected to increase by more than 60% by 2050 [3, 4]. According to the 2010 Global Burden of Disease Study by Chung et al., it is estimated that at least 33 million people worldwide had atrial fibrillation as of 2010, and data analysis showed that from 1990 to 2010, the prevalence and incidence of atrial fibrillation in both men and women after age adjustment increased significantly [4]. The prevalence of atrial fibrillation in Europe is also high, with studies showing that there will be about 9 million cases by 2016, and the number of patients with atrial fibrillation in Europe will increase significantly in the next few decades and may even increase 1-fold between 2010 ~ 2060 [4].

2.2 Causes of atrial fibrillation

There are many causes of atrial fibrillation, mainly coronary heart disease and myocardial diseases in developed countries, and rheumatic valvular heart disease in developing countries. A small percentage of atrial fibrillations with no clear causes is called isolated or idiopathic atrial fibrillation. Common causes are as follows:

1. Hypertension Patients with AF typically have other concomitant cardiovascular risk factors—hypertension being one of the commonly associated conditions with a prevalence of up to 90% in major clinical trials of AF [5]. The occurrence of atrial fibrillation is related to the abnormal electrophysiological of hypertrophic myocardium, hypertrophic myocardial ischemia, and hypertrophic myocardial fibrosis caused. Because of myocardial hypertrophy and fibrosis, decreased ventricular compliance and increased atrial pressure, thereby atrial fibrillation was induced by atrial electrophysiology disorder.

2. Coronary heart disease In coronary angiography shows that there is 0.6 to 0.8% of atrial fibrillation in obvious coronary artery stenosis, and atrial fibrillation in acute myocardial infarction accounted for 10 ~ 15%.

3. Rheumatic heart disease remains a common cause of atrial fibrillation, particularly mitral stenosis with insufficiency. Among them, 41% of patients with mitral stenosis have atrial fibrillation, and aortic valve lesions have a small chance of atrial fibrillation. The average age at which patients develop atrial fibrillation is about 37 years, mostly women.

4. Heart disease of pulmonary origin The incidence of atrial fibrillation in lung disease is reported as 4–5%. Paroxysmal causes are related to recurrent pulmonary infections, chronic hypoxia, acidosis, and electrolyte abnormalities.

5. Congenital heart disease In congenital heart disease, atrial fibrillation is seen in cases when atrial septal defect is present.

6. Cardiomyopathy Atrial fibrillation can occur in various types of cardiomyopathies, and the incidence is between 10–50%, more common in adults, and can also occur in children. Primary congestive cardiomyopathy is predominant, accounting for about 20%.

7. Hyperthyroidism Atrial fibrillation is one of the main symptoms of hyperthyroidism, the incidence of atrial fibrillation in hyperthyroid patients is 15% ~ 20%, and the elderly with hyperthyroidism may have organic damage to the myocardium prone to chronic atrial fibrillation. Atrial fibrillation may be the first presentation in some patients.

8. Preexcitation syndrome also called Wolff-Parkinson-White (WPW). It should be mentioned that preexcitation syndrome and atrial fibrillation are more likely to occur together. The literature reports that the probability of atrial fibrillation and preexcitation syndrome occurring simultaneously is about 12 ~ 18% [6]. The incidence of atrial fibrillation with ventricular preexcitation is generally considered to be age-dependent, rarely in children, and higher in older patients.

2.3 Mechanism of atrial fibrillation

Atrial fibrillation has undergone theories such as "multiple microwave reentry," "rapid release of impulse foci," "local venous foci driven with fibrillation-like conduction," and the recent "pulmonary vein-left atrial reentry." Single or paired premature atrial beats or tachycardia due to ectopic focal rapid impulse discharge is one of the most common triggers of atrial fibrillation, and multiple wave reentrants are the main mechanism by which atrial fibrillation is maintained.

2.3.1 Myocardial fibrosis

Studies have confirmed that the pathological basis of the pathogenesis of atrial fibrillation is related to myocardial fibrosis and the reduction of atrial muscle tissue content, the left atrium enlarges when atrial fibrillation occurs, aggravates myocardial interstitial fibrosis, reduces the content of healthy atrial muscle tissue and the number of cells, remodeling the extracellular matrix is obvious, and the difference in the refractory period of atrial muscle is significant. The dilated atria activate the RAAS system, which together contributes to the onset and maintenance of atrial fibrillation.

2.3.2 Molecular biological mechanisms

Atrial fibrillation is a progressive condition that begins with paroxysmal and becomes persistent or permanent. Structural and molecular biological changes that occur in the central atrium of the course of the disease are called atrial remodeling. Early changes are manifested as changes in electrophysiology and ion channel characteristics, also known as electro remodeling. Electro remodeling, predominantly reduced L-type calcium channels, predisposes to atrial muscle fibrillation [7]. In the late stage of atrial reconstruction, it is manifested as fibrosis, starch deposition, apoptosis, and other changes in the tissue structure of the atrium, which is called remodeling. Ultrastructural changes in atrial myocytes and fibrosis of the myocardial interstitium, as well as redistribution of collagen fibers, manifested as atrial myocyte hypertrophy, perinuclear glycogen accumulation, atrial myocyte lysis, and changes in atrial connexin at the cellular level. At the molecular level, it is manifested as degradation of structural proteins and contractile proteins, disordered arrangement of slit junction proteins, and degradation of ion channel proteins. Atrial structure remodeling is macroscopically manifested as atrial enlargement.

2.3.3 Molecular genetic mechanism

In 1928, Wolff and White observed that the incidence of atrial fibrillation has a familial tendency to cluster, and there have been reports of familial atrial fibrillation in China since 1979. Seen in: (1) Gene variation on chromosome 11: Chen Yihan et al. [8] reported in the journal science that the S140G mutation of the KCNQ1 gene

DOI: http://dx.doi.org/10.5772/intechopen.113163

in a Chinese family line of atrial fibrillation was located, and the KCNQ1 gene was localized in the chromosome 11pl5.5 region. With the application of gene correlation analysis and gene mapping cloning technology, more and more studies have found that the onset of atrial fibrillation is related to the polymorphism of multiple genes. Gai [9] and other scholars found that TIMP2-418G > C gene polymorphisms are associated with the incidence of atrial fibrillation in Han hypertensive heart disease people. CMA1 polymorphisms may be associated with AF, and the rs1800875 GG genotype might be a susceptibility factor for AF in Chinese people [10].

2.3.4 Oxidative stress

In recent years, oxidative stress has been considered to be one of the important mechanisms for the development of atrial fibrillation, and reactive oxygen species (ROS) are produced by oxidative metabolism. The prevalence and incidence of atrial fibrillation have been found to be related to the redox potential of the oxidative stress markers called glutathione and cysteine, with a 10% increase in the prevalence of atrial fibrillation [11]. In addition to the electrical remodeling stimulated by the mechanisms described, ROS have also been demonstrated to contribute to atria structural remodeling. Researchers from Slovakia showed that hydroxyl radicals can alter the myofibrillar protein structure and function, promoting myocardial injury and further contributing to the formation of a fertile substrate for the development of arrhythmias. In addition to the electrical remodeling stimulated by the mechanisms described, ROS have also been demonstrated to contribute to atria structural remodeling. Other studies have shown [12] that RyR2 is oxidized in the atria of patients with chronic atrial fibrillation compared to individuals with sinus rhythm, and changes in RyR2 and production of mitochondrial ROS create a vicious cycle in the development of AF.

2.3.5 Inflammation and atrial fibrillation

Li et al. have found that elevated serum CRP levels are positively correlated with atrial fibrillation [13]. Elevated plasma CRP concentrations have not in themselves been shown to increase the risk of atrial fibrillation, and CCL2 values obtained suggest that inflammation may be the result of AF [14]. Recent studies have shown that the P wave dispersion and hs-CRP levels of paroxysmal atrial fibrillation are significantly higher than those in the control group [15]. In addition, inflammation promotes thrombotic load, stimulates platelet formation, increases thrombin sensitivity, and promotes the transformation of fibrinogen.

3. Clinical symptoms of atrial fibrillation

The clinical manifestations of atrial fibrillation are diverse and can be symptomatic or asymptomatic. This is true even for the same patient. The symptoms of atrial fibrillation depend on a variety of factors, including ventricular rate at the time of attack, cardiac function, concomitant conditions, duration of atrial fibrillation, and sensitivity to perceived symptoms. Most patients experience palpitations, dyspnea, chest pain, thinness, and dizziness. Some people with atrial fibrillation have no symptoms and are only detected during a physical examination or by chance serious complications of atrial fibrillation such as stroke, embolism, or heart failure. Some patients have symptoms of left ventricular dysfunction, which may be secondary to atrial fibrillation with a persistent rapid ventricular rate. Syncope is uncommon but is a serious complication that often suggests sinus node dysfunction and atrioventricular conduction abnormalities or post-thrombosis exfoliation during atrial fibrillation transition.

4. Classification of atrial fibrillation

According to the time and characteristics of the onset, atrial fibrillation can be divided into primary atrial fibrillation, paroxysmal atrial fibrillation, persistent atrial fibrillation, long-term persistent atrial fibrillation, or permanent atrial fibrillation (Eur Heart J 2010, 31: 2369–2429), which is a commonly used classification method in clinical practice.

5. Treatment of atrial fibrillation

Rhythm control and ventricular rate control are the two major strategies for the treatment of atrial fibrillation. Theoretically, it is better to restore and maintain sinus rhythm, but it should be appropriate for individual and disease-specific treatment, and it is necessary to fully weigh the benefits of conversion to patients and the disadvantages of antiarrhythmic drugs. Drugs remain the first-line treatment of choice for controlling heart rhythm and ventricular rate.

The main principles of atrial fibrillation treatment are: (1) try to find the basic causes of atrial fibrillation for treatment, such as correcting heart valve lesions, correcting hypotension, improving heart function, alleviating myocardial ischemia, controlling hyperthyroidism, etc., (2) elimination of predisposing factors, conversion, and maintenance of sinus rhythm, (3) prevention of recurrence, (4) control ventricular rate, and (5) prevent embolic complications, reduce the disability rate, improve the quality of life of patients, and prolong life.

5.1 Treatment of causes

Treatment of the cause of atrial fibrillation is critical, and aggressive treatment of primary heart disease is the easiest way to convert atrial fibrillation to sinus rhythm and maintain it for a long time. Even if the cause cannot be cured, it is important to resolve the hemodynamic abnormality. In cases of coronary heart disease, hypertension, cardiomyopathy, etc., such as improvement of myocardial ischemia, correction of heart failure, good blood pressure control, the chance of atrial fibrillation conversion is increased, and sinus rhythm can be maintained for a long time. In patients with mitral valve stenosis and atrial fibrillation in rheumatic heart disease, many patients are able to maintain sinus rhythm long after cardioversion after surgery to remove the cause.

5.2 Upstream treatment

Drugs for upstream treatment include angiotensin-converting enzyme inhibitors (ACEI) and angiotensin II receptor blockers (ARBs), aldosterone antagonists, statins, polyunsaturated fatty acid (PUFA), and LCZ696. It can reduce myocardial fibrosis and heterogeneity in the electrical activity of the atrial myocardia. Studies have shown that ACE inhibitors and ARBs can prevent the shortening of the effective refractory period of the atrium, inhibit the early remodeling of the atria [16], and inhibit the occurrence of atrial fibrillation. On the one hand, it may be related to reversal of atrial structural remodeling and electrical remodeling, and inhibition of atrial fibrillation may be achieved through anti-inflammatory and antioxidant effects [17]. Mariscalco G [18] et al. studied 530 patients undergoing cardiac surgery and found that preoperative supplementation with ω-3 PUFA may reduce the incidence of early postoperative AF, but not the incidence of late AF. Studies have shown LCZ696 [19] can simultaneously regulate the natriuretic peptide system and RAAS system, curb the deterioration of heart failure and atrial fibrillation, and combat the pathophysiological changes, such as myocardial remodeling.

5.3 Drug therapy

Medical treatment of atrial fibrillation includes cardioversion, control of ventricular rate, and anticoagulation. This chapter focuses on drug cardioversion.

5.3.1 Drug cardioversion

At present, the drugs commonly used in domestic clinical practice are Class Ic and Class III antiarrhythmic drugs, including Flecainide, Propafenone, Morecizidine, Iblit, vinacalan, dronedarone, ranolazine, and ivabradine.

5.3.1.1 Indications for drug cardioversion

(1) persistent atrial fibrillation is less than half a year, or there is no blood clot in the atrium confirmed by ultrasonography, (2) for patients with paroxysmal atrial fibrillation, it can be treated during the onset of atrial fibrillation or between episodes, and (3) maintain sinus rhythm with drugs after electrical cardioversion.

5.3.1.2 Drug selection

The clinical drug selection principles that should be observed when performing drug reversion in atrial fibrillation are:

1. Paroxysmal atrial fibrillation with or without organic heart disease (but not coronary heart disease and left ventricular hypertrophy) can choose Class Ic antiarrhythmic drugs, such as propafenone, followed by sotalol and ibutilide. If it is still ineffective, amiodarone is an option, but it may also be preferred.

2. Patients with organic heart disease or heart failure: Amiodarone is the drug of choice.

3. Patients with coronary heart disease (including acute myocardial infarction) and atrial fibrillation: Amiodarone should be preferred and sotalol should be selected.

4. Vagus nerve-mediated atrial fibrillation: Amiodarone, amiodarone and flecainide, can also be used.

It should be noted that patients with organic heart disease and atrial fibrillation, especially with coronary heart disease and heart failure, should try to use amiodarone and sotalol, and avoid use the Class Ia (quinidine) and Ic (propafenone) drugs.

The success rate of atrial fibrillation conversion by injecting amiodarone is 34% ~ 69%, and the success rate of oral conversion is 15 ~ 40%, but its clinical application is limited due to its serious side effects.

Intravenous propafenone can convert atrial fibrillation, which has a good effect on recent occurrences, is characterized by fewer adverse reactions, and should be used with caution in patients with organic heart disease.

Recent studies have shown that Ibutilide is a new fast-acting safe class III antiarrhythmic drug with unique ion channel activity. It has intravenous medication that can effectively terminate atrial tachycardia, atrial flutter, and atrial fibrillation, and has the characteristics of fast onset, high efficacy, and fast metabolism. In particular, the success rate of atrial flutter and atrial fibrillation conversion within 2 weeks is significantly higher than that of chronic atrial flutter and atrial fibrillation. Intravenous administration of Ibutilide 1 ~ 2 mg takes effect in 30 to 40 min. Compared with electrical cardioversion, there is no need for anesthesia, which is more convenient and safer to use, and there is no need to adjust the dose for patients with liver and kidney dysfunction. Zhao Jingjing et al. [20] showed that ibutilide combined with radiofrequency ablation has a good therapeutic effect on elderly patients with atrial fibrillation, which can improve the conversion rate after treatment, reduce the recurrence rate after surgery, and reduce the damage to the myocardium. As a novel potassium channel blocker, Ibutilide can inhibit the delayed rectified potassium (Ikr) current that is rapidly activated during repolarization, which is different from other class III antiarrhythmic drugs, Ibutilide also has the effect of promoting slow Na + influx and Ca2+ influx during the plateau phase, counteracting the effect of partial K+ outflow, and prolonging the plateau phase of cardiomyocytes action potential. Prolong the time course of myocardial action potential, prolong the QT interval and effective refractory period, and affect the entire repolarization process. The effect of Ibutilide on the atria is more obvious than that of the ventricle, its effect is 10 times stronger and can extend the effective refractory period of the atrial muscle by 90–110%, Ibutilide will become an important drug for the treatment of atrial tachycardia, atrial flutter, and atrial fibrillation in the future, bringing benefits to patients with atrial arrhythmia. It takes effect about 1 hour after intravenous injection, and its effect of conversion to atrial flutter is better than that of atrial fibrillation. For long-term atrial fibrillation, the literature reports that about 4% of patients develop torsion ventricular tachycardia after injection, and it is more likely to occur in women, so it should be performed under supervision and the post-medication monitoring time should not be less than 5 hours.

At present, quinidine and procainamide are rarely used for conversion, mainly due to their serious adverse effects, and the effect of disopyramide and sotalol conversion to atrial fibrillation is uncertain.

In recent years, new drugs have gradually occupied a certain position in the conversion of atrial fibrillation, such as donedarone and venakalan have a good effect on the conversion of atrial fibrillation.

Dronedarone is a new class III antiarrhythmic drug, its structure is similar to amiodarone, but does not contain iodine, few extracardiac adverse reactions, and the usual dose is 400 mg twice a day. It can reduce the hospitalization rate of cardiovascular disease and arrhythmia mortality rate in patients with atrial fibrillation, but the effectiveness of maintaining sinus rhythm is not as good as amiodarone, guidelines recommend the first-line drug for nonpermanent atrial fibrillation of mild or nonorganic heart disease, but contraindicated in NYHA grade III ~ IV heart failure.

Vernakalant, the first atrial selective atrial fibrillation treatment drug currently on the market, acts on both sodium and potassium channels. The drug is metabolized by the liver pigment P4502D6 isoenzyme, with a half-life of about 4 ~ 8 hours, and is not affected by age, kidney function, and other drugs. The drug has a low incidence of side effects. Vinakalan is currently approved by the European Union for the relapse of adult patients with newly developed atrial fibrillation cardioversion therapy. (onset ≤7 days in nonsurgical patients and ≤ 3 days in postoperative patients).

5.3.2 Combined application of drugs

The combined application of two different antiarrhythmic drugs has an accumulation of effects, a dose reduction, and a decrease in the incidence of adverse reactions, but attention must be paid to their mutual effects. Clinically, β receptor blockers, non-dihydropyridine calcium channel blockers, digoxin, and amiodarone are used to control the ventricular rate of atrial arrhythmias and strive to convert to sinus rhythm. For example, small doses of digitalis combined with β blockers to control the ventricular rate in patients with atrial fibrillation. Amiodarone is safe and effective for atrial arrhythmias in patients with structural heart disease and heart failure due to its weak negative inotropic effect.

Author details

Taomin Su[1*], Pan Liu[2], Qin Shi[2], Yan Wang[1] and Ying Zhou[1]

1 Xuhui Hospital, Fudan University, China

2 Gongli Hospital, Pudong New District, Shanghai, China

*Address all correspondence to: sutaomin_2020@sina.com

IntechOpen

© 2023 The Author(s). Licensee IntechOpen. This chapter is distributed under the terms of the Creative Commons Attribution License (http://creativecommons.org/licenses/by/3.0), which permits unrestricted use, distribution, and reproduction in any medium, provided the original work is properly cited. (cc) BY

References

[1] Collins D, Leeder DB. Pathogenesis of atrial fibrillation and implications for treatment. Australian Veterinary Practitioner. 2012;**42**(2):256-261

[2] Zhang J et al. Epidemiology of atrial fibrillation: Geographic/ecological risk factors, age, sex, genetics. Cardiac Electrophysiology Clinics. 2021;**13**(1):1-23

[3] Chugh SS et al. Worldwide epidemiology of atrial fibrillation: A global burden of disease 2010 study. Circulation. 2014;**129**(8):837-847

[4] Krijthe BP et al. Projections on the number of individuals with atrial fibrillation in the European Union, from 2000 to 2060. European Heart Journal. 2013;**34**(35):2746-2751

[5] Gue YX, Lip G. Hypertension and atrial fibrillation: Closing a virtuous circle. PLoS Medicine. 2021;**18**(6):e1003598

[6] Centurión OA et al. Mechanisms for the genesis of paroxysmal atrial fibrillation in the Wolff Parkinson-white syndrome: Intrinsic atrial muscle vulnerability vs. electrophysiological properties of the accessory pathway. Europace. 2008;**10**(3):294-302

[7] Li ML et al. Research of L-type Ca^{2+} channel current in atrial myocytes of patients with chronic atrial fibrillation. Zhonghua Xin Xue Guan Bing Za Zhi. 2006;**34**(4):308-311

[8] Chen YH et al. KCNQ1 gain-of-function mutation in familial atrial fibrillation. Science. 2003;**299**(5604):251-254

[9] Gai X et al. MMP-2 and TIMP-2 gene polymorphisms and susceptibility to atrial fibrillation in Chinese Han patients with hypertensive heart disease. Clinica Chimica Acta. 2010;**411**(9-10):719-724

[10] Zhou D et al. Association between chymase gene polymorphisms and atrial fibrillation in Chinese Han population. BMC Cardiovascular Disorders. 2019;**19**(1):321

[11] Samman TA et al. Association between oxidative stress and atrial fibrillation. Heart Rhythm. 2017;**14**(12):1849-1855

[12] Xie W et al. Mitochondrial oxidative stress promotes atrial fibrillation. Scientific Reports. 2015;**5**:11427

[13] Li X et al. C-reactive protein and atrial fibrillation: Insights from epidemiological and Mendelian randomization studies. Nutrition, Metabolism, and Cardiovascular Diseases. 2022;**32**(6):1519-1527

[14] Alegret JM et al. The relevance of the association between inflammation and atrial fibrillation. European Journal of Clinical Investigation. 2013;**43**(4):324-331

[15] Tsioufis C et al. Relationships of CRP and P wave dispersion with atrial fibrillation in hypertensive subjects. American Journal of Hypertension. 2010;**23**(2):202-207

[16] Hagiwara N. Inflammation and atrial fibrillation. Circulation Journal. 2010;**74**(2):246-247

[17] Hirayama Y et al. Long-term effects of upstream therapy on paroxysmal atrial fibrillation in patients without overt heart diseases. International Heart Journal. 2009;**50**(2):141-151

[18] Mariscalco G et al. Preoperative n-3 polyunsaturated fatty acids are associated with a decrease in the incidence of early atrial fibrillation following cardiac surgery. Angiology. 2010;**61**(7):643-650

[19] Tsutsui H et al. Efficacy and safety of sacubitril/valsartan (LCZ696) in Japanese patients with chronic heart failure and reduced ejection fraction: Rationale for and design of the randomized, double-blind PARALLEL-HF study. Journal of Cardiology. 2017;**70**(3):225-231

[20] Jingjing Z, Weifeng S. Clinical analysis of ibutilide combined with radiofrequency ablation in the treatment of atrial fibrillation in the elderly. Journal of Aerospace Medicine. 2022;**33**(11):1305-1308

Section 3

Automated External Defibrillation

Chapter 5

AED: Optimal Use of Automated External Defribilators in BLS and ILS

Tudor Ovidiu Popa, Mihaela Corlade-Andrei, Paul Nedelea, Emilian Manolescu, Alexandra Hauta and Diana Cimpoesu

Abstract

The use of Automatic External Defibrillators (AED) present in public access defibrillation programs (PAD) in cardiopulmonary resuscitation (CPR) is a challenge in the effective treatment of cardiac arrest, especially for adult patients. It is already known that the majority of adult cases of out-of-hospital cardiac arrest arise from ventricular fibrillation (VF). The most important factor in determining survival from VF is the time from collapse to defibrillation. If laypersons are trained to perform Basic Life Support (BLS) and to attempt defibrillation using an automatic external defibrillator before the emergency medical services arrive, the survival rate of an out-of-hospital cardiac arrest can be increased. In many countries, the number of public access AEDs has increased but implementation of AED use and CPR performed by public bystanders has not been sufficiently frequent. In fact, only a minority of individuals demonstrate sufficient knowledge and willingness to operate an AED, suggesting that the public is not yet sufficiently prepared. It is also very important to support the permanent campaign of training as many laypersons, starting from school, to properly use such defibrillators in public places. Considering these facts, PAD is an effective way and may be a cost-effective way to improve outcomes in cardiac arrest.

Keywords: automatic external Defibrilator (AED), BLS, ILS, defibrillation, CPR, bystanders, cardiac arrest, education

1. Introduction

Defibrillation is an essential link in the chain of survival in case of ventricular fibrillation (VF) and pulseless ventricular tachycardia (pVT).

For every minute that passes without applying defibrillation, the chance of the patient to respond to this maneuver is decreasing by 7–10%, decreasing also the chance of surviving.

Automated external defibrillators (AEDs) are portable smart life savings devices, designed to administer the necessary treatment for people experiencing sudden cardiac arrest, a medical condition in which the heart stops beating suddenly and unexpectedly when VF or pVT is present.

Public access AEDs can be found in airports, community centers, schools, government buildings, and other crowded public locations. They are intended to be used by lay people who have received minimal or no training.

AEDs are a type of computerized defibrillator that automatically analyzes the heart rhythm in people who are suffering cardiac arrest. When appropriate, it delivers an external electric shock to the heart muscle, the goal being to restore its normal sinusal rhythm.

The combination of cardiopulmonary resuscitation (CPR) and early defibrillation is effective in saving lives when used in the first few minutes following a collapse from sudden cardiac arrest, if the victim presents a cardiac arrest rhythm that requires defibrillation, like ventricular fibrillation or ventricular tachycardia without a pulse.

The AED devices include some accessories, such as pads (electrodes), that are necessary for the AED to detect and interpret a person's heart rhythm and also necessary to deliver an external electric shock if it is needed. There are two main types of AEDs: public access and professional use.

Professional use AEDs are used by first responders, such as emergency medical technicians (EMTs) and paramedics, who receive additional AED training.

Automated defibrillators analyze the heart's rhythm, and if an abnormal heart rhythm is detected, that requires a shock, then the device prompts the user to press a button to deliver a defibrillation shock.

A defibrillator should be used as soon as possible when a person is found in cardiac arrest. CPR should be performed until a defibrillator is brought on the scene.

2. Defibrillation

Defibrillation is an essential link in the chain of survival, in the case of cardiac arrest produced by ventricular fibrillation (VF) and pulseless ventricular tachycardia (pVT). After the onset of cardiac arrest, the circulation is absent and the hypoxic brain injury begins to appear after 3 minutes, if in this interval nobody starts to perform chest compressions.

Defibrillation maneuver can stop cardiac arrest produced by VF/pVT by applying an external electric asynchronous shock, at up to 5 seconds after its application, by depolarizing the myocardium and restoring normal electrical activity, compatible with the presence of a pulse.

Although defibrillation is the most important in the management of patients with shockable rhythms (VF/pVT), also continuous, high quality uninterrupted external chest compressions are required to optimize the chances of successful resuscitation [1–3].

The success of defibrillation depends on the transmission of the energy to the myocardium and the following conditions are involved:

- The position of the electrodes (pads);
- Transthoracic impedance (depending on the size of the electrodes, the contact between skin and electrodes, contact point pressure, breathing phase);
- Delivered energy;
- Dimensions of the victim's body (body impedance).

In the case of cardiac arrest produced in the pre-hospital, the emergency medical personnel must ensure good quality resuscitation throughout the interval of bringing, applying, and charging the defibrillator. A predetermined duration (for example, two minutes) of CPR before rhythm analysis and shock delivery is no longer recommended, the defibrillator should be used as soon as this is available.

During resuscitation, different types of defibrillators are used depending on the place where the cardiac arrest occurred, the training of the resuscitation team, technical possibilities, and economic resources [2, 4, 5].

Automatic external defibrillation can be used by bystanders, paramedics, non-medical personnel, or personnel with medical training who intervene in situations of cardiorespiratory arrest out of the hospital and in some situations in the hospital. Regarding manual defibrillation, this is performed only by medically trained personnel who have the theoretical and practical knowledge necessary to recognize and defibrillate correctly a shockable rhythm [2, 4, 5].

3. Use of automated external defibrillator

AEDs are safe and effective when used by lay people without or with minimal knowledge of defibrillation.

AEDs make defibrillation possible with many minutes before the arrival of qualified medical help. Resuscitators should focus on voice commands as soon as they begin, especially resuming CPR as soon as possible and minimizing the interruption of chest compressions.

Standard AEDs are suitable for use in children over 8 years of age. Pediatric self-adhesive paddles are used for children between 1 and 8 years old [1].

The use of the automatic external defibrillator by EMS in the pre-hospital settings.

In the case of out-of-hospital cardiac arrest, the emergency medical personnel must ensure good quality resuscitation during the entire interval of bringing, applying, and loading the defibrillator. For emergency medical services that have implemented a predetermined period of chest compressions before defibrillation, due to the lack of convincing data, it is reasonable for these services to continue this practice [1, 2].

Below is the guide for using the AED which does not require knowledge of electrocardiography, physiopathology of ventricular fibrillation, or defibrillation energy.

Instead, there is essential knowledge about the device and how to use it, following verbal instructions, knowledge of safety measures in defibrillation, and CPR measures.

The device is equipped with self-adhesive pads, which are placed above the level of the apex of the heart and on the right, subclavicular, or antero-posterior presternal and interscapular.

For patients with implantable medical devices (pacemaker for permanent electrical cardiostimulation, implantable defibrillator), electrodes of defibrillation will be placed at a distance from the device (at least 8 cm) or will use an alternative positioning (antero-lateral, antero-posterior).

Also, the transdermal patches should be removed and cleaned the area before applying the self-adhesive electrodes.

Defibrillation should be performed with minimal interruption of chest compressions (less than 5 seconds, actual recommendation being 3 seconds). Thus, the pause in chest compression can be reduced to less than 5 seconds by continuing chest

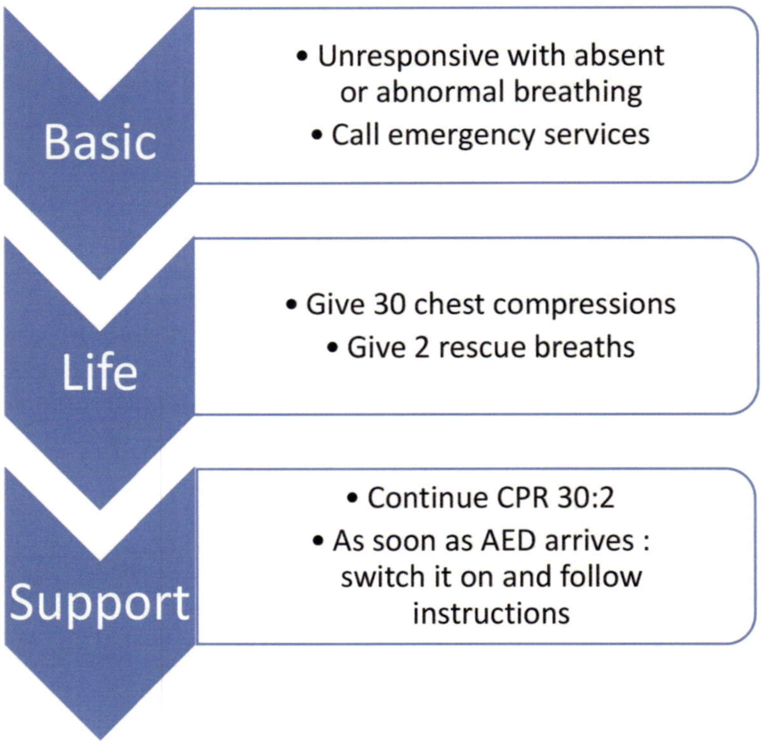

Figure 1.
BLS algorithm. (https://www.cprguidelines.eu/assets/posters/BLS-Algorithms-portrait.pdf).

compressions during charging of the defibrillator and by effective coordination of the resuscitation team, and minimizing pause.

After each schock, immediately resuming chest compressions is extremely important, this strategy should be applied after each shock administration.

In **Figure 1**, we present the BLS and AED algorithm steps from the Basic Life Support algorithm, accordingly to European Resuscitation Council Guideline 2021.

4. Types of energy used in defibrillation

Defibrillation requires the release of sufficient energy to depolarize a critical mass in the myocardium, to stop the chaotic electrical activity and to allow the normal activity of the natural pacemaker to be resumed.

The use of monophasic defibrillators for almost 30 years has brought many benefits, but it also allowed the myocardial injury to be highlighted, produced by the passage of the defibrillation current through the heart.

The monophasic defibrillators, which currently are no longer produced, but continue to be in use, release a unipolar current, which crosses the heart in one direction. There are two types of monophasic current: attenuated sinusoidal current and truncated exponential current.

Modern biphasic defibrillators are designed to deliver a current that crosses the myocardium in both directions: positive and negative. There are also two types of current delivered by this defibrillator: truncated biphasic current and rectilinear biphasic current.

DOI: http://dx.doi.org/10.5772/intechopen.111907

The advantages of biphasic defibrillators are:

- requires less energy for successful defibrillation;
- have smaller capacitors and batteries are smaller;
- they are lighter and more convenient to transport;
- biphasic shocks with energy <200 J have a higher success rate in VF/pVT conversion than 360 J monophasic shocks.

Clinical studies have proven the superiority of defibrillation with defibrillators biphasic, the myocardial injury being minimal, and the efficiency maximal.

5. The automatic external defibrillator

The automatic external defibrillator is a computerized device with the ability to recognize automatically a heart rhythm that requires an external electric shock and to give the indication to apply the external electric shock (in the case of VF/pVT). The sensitivity of the device to recognize a shockable rhythm is very high, AEDs are designed such that they have a very high specificity (>99%) in detecting shockable rhythms.

The device is provided with self-adhesive electrodes (pads), which are placed anteriorly at the apex of the heart and at right, subclavicular position, or antero-posterior (presternal and interscapular, if the situation requires this, for example, wounds present an apex level). To facilitate the positioning of the pads over the chest, on each of them is drawn the place where should be applied.

The presence of a transdermal drug patch on the patient's chest may prevent good contact and may cause electrical arcing and burns if self-adhesive pads are placed over them. Place the pads in an alternative position that avoids the patch or remove the patches and dry the skin area. If an implantable device is present(pacemaker), the pads should be placed at least 8 cm distance.

According to the new recommendations of the Advance Life Support 2021 published by the European Resuscitation Council, defibrillation must be performed with minimal interruption, this should be performed in less than 3 seconds [2–4].

The protocol for using the automatic/semi-automatic defibrillator:

1. Open the device
2. Connect the device to the patient by applying the self-adhesive electrodes on the patient's chest and attach the electrodes to the device. During steps 1 and 2 perform high-quality chest compressions.
3. Set ANALYSIS mode, and interrupt chest compressions during analysis.
4. Shock. If the rhythm of the cardiac arrest is a shockable VF/pVT, the AED indicates the need to apply the shock and automatically charges 150-360 J. Announce with a loud voice the application of the shock and check that no one is in contact with the patient.

Immediately after applying the external shock, restart CPR (30 chest compressions: 2 ventilations). Repeat these steps after 2 minutes of CPR if VF/pVT is present [1, 2].

6. Use of AED in the hospital

In every medical facility should be available a defibrillator which can be used in maximum 3 minutes in case of a cardiac arrest occur in a patient. Depending on the partcularityes of each medical facility and the presence of the trained personnel this could be an AED or a manual defibrillator.

There are no published randomized clinical trials comparing the utility of AEDs and manual defibrillators in the hospital. Three observational studies have shown that there is no improvement in the survival of adult patients at discharge following a cardiac arrest when using an AED, compared to a manual defibrillator.

A large observational study showed that in-hospital use of AED was associated with lower survival compared to the one who were defibrillated with a manual defibrillator, suggesting that AED may cause delays in starting CPR or stopping chest compressions in patients with non-shockable rhythm. The goal is to attempt defibrillation within 3 minutes of collapse [1, 5].

According to the recommendations of the resuscitation guide of the European Council of Resuscitation, up to three successive external electric shocks can be used if ventricular fibrillation/pulseless ventricular tachycardia (VF/VT) occurs during cardiac catheterization or immediately in the postoperative period after cardiac surgery. This three shock strategy can also be considered in case of cardiac arrest assisted by VF/pVT when the patient is already monitored with a manual defibrillator or AED.

Throughout resuscitation and defibrillation, it is important to minimize the duration of the pre- and post-shock pauses, the continuity of chest compressions are recommended during defibrillator charging and rapid resumption of chest compressions after each defibrillation.

During resuscitation, different types of defibrillators are used, depending on multiple factors like the place where the cardiac arrest occurred, the training of the resuscitation team, but also the technical possibilities, the economic resources, and the health programs of each community.

Automated external defibrillation is used by paramedical staff, non-medical, or with medium medical training that intervenes in situations of cardiorespiratory arrest in the prehospital settings, but also in some situations even in the hospital.

In **Table 1**, we present the guidance for using AED:

Stages of use	Details of operations
1. Identify cardiac arrest	1. Start CPR Ask someone to bring the nearest defibrillator
2. Open/Start the defibrilator	2. Open the device and follow guidance from the device (spoken or visual) Continue CPR
3. Connecting the device	3. Connect the device to the patient • apply the self-adhesive electrodes on the patient's chest • attach the electrodes to the device Continue CPR

Stages of use	Details of operations
4. Mode setting ANALYZE	4. Analysis • notify the nurse and check if the patient is not in contact with another person • press the ANALYZE button Stop CPR
5. SHOCK	5. Shock delivery0. If FV/pVT is present, the device indicates the need to apply the shock and it automatically charges to 150–360 J. • announce the application of the shock • check again that no one is in contact with the patient • press the SHOCK button after the device is charged. Immediately after applying the shock, resume CPR (30 compressions/2 ventilations). Repeat these steps after 2 min. of CPR as long as VF/pVT is present.

Table 1.
Guidelines for using AED in hospital.

7. Recommendation for semi-automated defibrillator

Semi-automated defibrillators are more complex devices that can be utilized in two modes, as an AED or as a manual defibrillator, depending on the medical personnel.

Manual defibrillation should only be performed by medical personnel, personnel who have the necessary theoretical and practical knowledge in recognition of a shockable rhythm.

Manual defibrillation involves, on the part of the operator:

- Identification of heart rhythm.
- Selection of energy, charging and applying shocks with the indicated energy;
- It can also be used to apply synchronous electric shock (cardioversion).

It is recommended to use self-adhesive electrodes for the defibrillation!

Safety rules:

- Never hold both paddles of the defibrillator in the same hand!
- If the patient is placed on a wet or conductive surface, move the patient to a safe space and dry the patient's chest before delivering the shock!
- Take care that no rescuer accidentally touches directly or indirectly, the patient at the time of shock delivery. Is recommended to use the formula "Attention, I'm defibrillating!"or "Clear!!"!
- Remove the oxygen sources from the defibrillation area (at least 1 meter)!

Defibrillation technique:

A single shock will be applied after every two minutes of resuscitation maneuvers:

- The older models of external defibrillators delivered a monophasic type of waveform. Biphasic defibrillation alternates the direction of the pulses, requires a low level of energy necessary for successful defibrillation, and decreases the risk of myocardial damage.

The first, as well as the following monophasic shocks will be delivered with 360 J;

- In the case of biphasic defibrillators, the first shock will be 150–200 J, the following 200 J, depending on the device up to 360 J;
- The shock will be immediately followed by CPR 30:2 for 2 minutes, without assessment of rhythm or central pulse immediately after administration of the shock. After defibrillation attempts, the majority of patients remain pulseless for at least 2 minutes, even if the defibrillation was successful and restored electrical activity at heart level, the recommendation is to immediately resume chest compressions for 2 minutes following each attempted defibrillation.
- After 2 min. of CPR, if VF/pVT persists, a new one shock will be applied; there is no recommendation for a maximum number of shocks within resuscitation, they will be delivered as long are necessary, if cardiac rhythm assessment performed after 2 minute of CPR identify VF/pVT;
- cardiac rhythm assessment will be done quickly after every 2 minutes of CPR, and evaluation of the central pulse only in the event of the appearance of a rhythm that could suggest the presence of pulse;
- If during the 2 min. of CPR after the shock, appear a rhythm compatible with the presence of spontaneous circulation, chest compressions will not be interrupted unless the victim also presents vital signs like (cough, spontaneous movements);
- If defibrillation restores the patient's circulation and VF/pVT occurs again, defibrillation will be resumed with the energy that was previously successful.

Manual defibrillation protocol:

- VF/pVT is identified on the defibrillator monitor;
- The correct energy level is selected;
- Charge the paddles/pads after they have been applied to the patient's chest;
- People around are warned: "Attention, shock!", "Clear!!";
- Visually check the area;
- The heart rate is checked once again on the monitor;
- The external electric shock is applied;
- Chest compressions and ventilations are initiated immediately, for 2 minutes,

8. Public access defibrillator programs

Regarding all the advantages of using AED in the first moments of cardiac arrest, there is a large consensus for the implementation of public access to defibrillators. Placement of AEDs in areas where a cardiac arrest can be recorded every 5 years is considered cost-effective and comparable to other medical interventions. Registering the AED for public access so the dispatcher can direct the resuscitator to a nearby AED can also help to optimize the response.

The effectiveness of AED use for victims at home is limited. The proportion of patients with FV is lower at home than in public places, however, the number of potential patients who could be treated at home is greater. Public access to defibrillators (PADs) rarely reaches patients at home.

Lay resuscitators performing CPR and directing to an AED can improve the chances of CPR and help reduce the time to defibrillation.

Universal AED Sign ILCOR has designed a simple and clear AED sign that can be recognized worldwide and is recommended to indicate the location of an AED.

Defibrillation programs with public access have the role of improving survival after cardiac arrest if they are established in locations where a cardiac arrest is likely to occur.

Suitable places may include airports, train stations, theaters, and sports facilities. Approximately 80% of prehospital cardiac arrests occur in private or residential settings. This inevitably limits the overall impact that PAD programs can have on survival rates [2, 5].

AED should be placed in public places (airports, train stations, theaters, stadiums) where there is an increased risk of cardiac arrest occurring with VF/pVT due to the high density of adults and can be used in various technical variants in defibrillation programs for the population—public access defibrillation—PAD.

Within the public programs for defibrillation, ILCOR created a universal sign (**Figure 2**) to indicate the location of an AED, a sign that can be recognized at the international level.

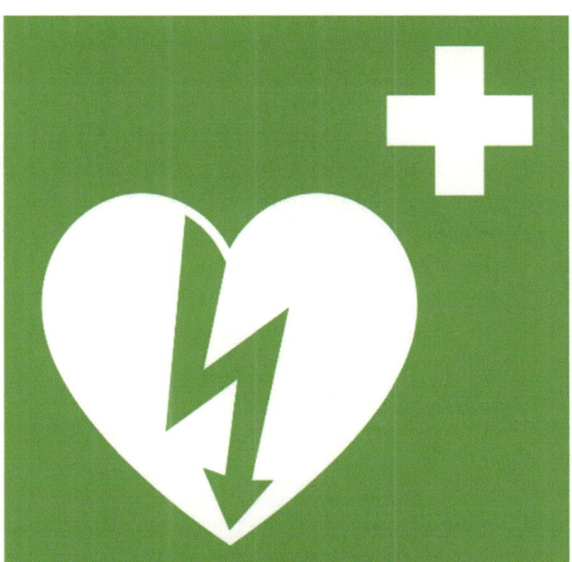

Figure 2.
ILCOR AED sign.

It is indicated that the entity or person who purchases the automatic external defibrillator to inform the emergency medical services about its existence; a physician should supervise it in order to ensure quality control and if there are persons responsible for using the automatic external defibrillator they should be trained on its correct use.

9. The factors that affect the success of defibrillation

Increased chest impedance reduces the level of energy delivered through the heart and decreases the chance of successful defibrillation. This is influenced by the contract between the pads and the skin, by the size of the pads, but also by the breathing phase, impedance being increased during inspiration(inhale) time.

The current recommendations are that the surface of the defibrillation electrode should be at least 150 cm^2, and the diameter should be 8–12 cm [1, 4, 6, 7].

10. Safety

The defibrillation attempt must be carried out without risk to the members of the resuscitation team. The main risk is represented by the accidentally direct or indirect electrocution of someone of the persons near the victim To minimize this risk, the best solution is to use self-adhesive pads *versus* paddles and by wearing gloves by the members of the medical team [1, 4, 6].

If an external electrical asynchronous shock is administered to someone who is not in VF or pulseless VT, it is possible some time to be applied exactly during the relative refractory period. If a shock is administered at this vulnerable moment of electric activity of the heart, it is a high chance to induce VF. Because of this, the defibrillation should only be performed for patients who present VF or pulseless VT [1, 4].

11. Conclusions

Regarding the use of the AED, it is certain that to save a life you need to know minimal things that are very helpful even if you are not a person in the medical field. And if you know from where to bring the defibrillator to the victim, you are still part of the chain of survival because you help the person providing first aid to do his job quickly and save time for the victim's life.

The importance of the interaction between the medical dispatcher, the witness who initiates CPR, including resuscitation maneuvers and timely use of automatic external defibrillator should be stressed.

Essentially, the coordinated community response, which attracts these elements, is essential for improving patient survival, if patient installs cardiorespiratory arrest outside the hospital.

The witness who is trained in Basic Life Support techniques and is available, must assess the victim quickly to determine if the victim is unconscious and not breathing normally, and then to alert the emergency services immediately.

The interaction between the medical dispatcher, the witness initiating CPR and the use of an AED are the essential elements for improving survival in case of cardiac arrest outside the hospital.

The victim who is unresponsive and not breathing normally is in cardiac arrest and requires CPR.

Witnesses and medical dispatchers must suspect cardiac arrest in any patient presenting with seizures and should carefully assess whether the victim breathing normally or not.

Rescuers trained in CPR should combine chest compressions with ventilations.

Conducting high-quality CPR remains essential for the improvement of the results.

Trained rescuers should provide chest compressions with an adequate depth (of at least 5 cm, but not more than 6 cm), with a frequency of 100–120 compressions per min. After each compression allow the chest to return, minimize interruptions during compressions.

When the savior performs breaths/ventilations for 1 second perform insufflation with a sufficient volume to ensure the expansion of the victim's chest.

Chest compression ratio and ventilation is 30:2. Do not stop chest compressions for more than 10 seconds to achieve ventilation.

Defibrillation performed within 3–5 minutes from the debut of cardiac arrest may increase the survival rate by more than 50–70%.

Early defibrillation can be achieved by the rescuer who initiates CPR using the automatic defibrillator external.

AEDs should be implemented in all spaces and public areas where there is a high population density.

We stress again the importance of implementing national programs for Basic Life Support and AED, to give access to defibrillators to the general public population. With these programs, the time from collapse to defibrillation can be greatly reduced.

Conflict of interest

The authors declare no conflict of interest.

Author details

Tudor Ovidiu Popa[1,2], Mihaela Corlade-Andrei[1,2*], Paul Nedelea[1,2], Emilian Manolescu[1,2], Alexandra Hauta[1,2] and Diana Cimpoesu[1,2]

1 Emergency Medicine Department, University of Medicine and Pharmacy Grigore T. Popa, Iasi, Romania

2 Clinical County Hospital St. Spiridon – Emergency Department, Iasi, Romania

*Address all correspondence to: corladeandrei.mihaela@gmail.com

IntechOpen

© 2023 The Author(s). Licensee IntechOpen. This chapter is distributed under the terms of the Creative Commons Attribution License (http://creativecommons.org/licenses/by/3.0), which permits unrestricted use, distribution, and reproduction in any medium, provided the original work is properly cited. (cc) BY

References

[1] Perkins GD, Olasveengen TM, Maconochie I, Soar J, Wyllie J, Greif R, et al. European resuscitation council guidelines for resuscitation: 2017 update. Resuscitation. 2018;**123**:43-50

[2] Exel W, Peran D, Jiménez FC. Advanced Life Support: Provider Manual. Emile Vanderveldelaan, Belgium: European Resuscitation Council vzw; 2021

[3] Liddle R, Davies CS, Colquhoun M, Handley AJ. The automated external defibrillator. BMJ. 2003;**327**(7425):1216

[4] Soar J, Böttiger BW, Carli P, Couper K, Deakin CD, Djärv T, et al. European resuscitation council guidelines 2021: Adult advanced life support. Resuscitation. 2021;**161**:115-151

[5] Soar J, Nolan JP, Böttiger BW, Perkins GD, Lott C, Carli P, et al. European resuscitation council guidelines for resuscitation 2015: Section 3. Adult advanced life support. Resuscitation. 2015;**95**:100-147

[6] Knight BP. Basic principles and technique of external electrical cardioversion and defibrillation. In: Post TW editor. UpToDate. Waltham, MA: UpToDate; 2023 [Accessed on June 06, 2023]

[7] Cimpoesu D, Popa O, Corlade M, et al. Guidelines and Algoritms in Emergency Medicine. Iasi: UMF "Gr. T. Popa" Publishing House; 2019

Chapter 6

The Influence of Transthoracic Impedance on Electrical Cardioversion and Defibrillation: Current Data

Adam Pal-Jakab, Bettina Nagy, Boldizsar Kiss and Endre Zima

Abstract

Sudden cardiac death (SCD) is a leading cause of death globally, often caused by malignant ventricular arrhythmias. Rapid termination by direct current defibrillation (DF) is the best way to treat pulseless ventricular tachycardia and ventricular fibrillation. Atrial fibrillation (AF) is the most common sustained arrhythmia in clinical practice. External cardioversion (ECV) is an immediate, effective, and safe procedure for the treatment of arrhythmias with high ventricular rate, for example, AF. The success of both ECV and DF is dependent on the delivery of sufficient current, influenced by energy and transthoracic impedance (TTI). TTI depends on patient characteristics, and the exact factors affecting it are still a matter of debate. Influencing factors such as respiration phase, contact pressure, coupling agent, and total energy delivered are commonly identified. However, there are multiple studies with controversial results concerning the effect of age, gender, body mass index, hemoglobin concentration, the presence of chronic heart failure, and fluid accumulation as independent predictors of TTI. The review emphasizes refining energy dosage during ECV and while minimizing complications caused by an unnecessarily high energy delivery. The value of TTI should be predicted to optimize the energy dosage and the number of shocks for successful ECV and DF.

Keywords: transthoracic impedance, defibrillation, cardioversion, electric current, delivered energy

1. Introduction

1.1 Sudden cardiac arrest and atrial fibrillation

Sudden cardiac death (SCD) is a major cause of death worldwide and the third leading cause of death in Europe [1]. In the European Union, there are 155,000–343,000 estimated SCD cases annually, with an incidence rate of 48.6 per 100,000 inhabitants. The number of SCD cases accounts for approximately 70% of the total annual expected number of Out-of-Hospital Cardiac Arrest (OHCA) cases in the

IntechOpen

European Union [2]. In the United States, SCD accounts for 7–18% of all deaths, or between 185,000 and 450,000 fatalities annually [3, 4].

The electrophysiological causes of SCD include shockable rhythms such as ventricular tachycardia (VT), ventricular fibrillation (VF), and other nonshockable rhythms. Ventricular arrhythmia therapy and SCD prevention involve managing underlying and concomitant conditions and diseases while preventing acute and progressive worsening [5]. In most cases, pharmacological therapy only has not been shown to be effective therapy enough; therefore, the proper consideration and implementation of device and pharmacological therapy are of paramount importance in the management of ventricular arrhythmias. The most effective device-assisted method of treating malignant ventricular tachycardias is the rapid termination by direct current defibrillation (DF).

Atrial fibrillation is the most common sustained cardiac arrhythmia, with a prevalence of up to 4% in the population over 20 years old. Treatment options include both pharmacological and nonpharmacological methods. In hemodynamically unstable patients with atrial fibrillation, an emergency electrical cardioversion (ECV) should be the preferred choice, while in stable patients, antiarrhythmic drugs preceding ECV can also be attempted. The benefits of rhythm control therapy include improving hemodynamics and quality of life, as well as reducing the time in arrhythmia, therefore the risk of potential thromboembolism, beside pharmacological therapeutic measures [6].

The success of both ECV and DF is dependent on the delivery of sufficient current. Current is determined by energy and transthoracic impedance (TTI). TTI largely depends on the patient's characteristics, and the exact factors affecting it are still a matter of debate.

1.2 Relevance of the chapter

Accurate identification of the exact influencing factors of TTI may lead to an increase in the efficacy of ECV and DF while minimizing the risk of complications. Adjusting the delivered energy according to identified clinical variables that independently influence the thoracic electrical impedance and hence the trans-myocardial current might result in more adequate defibrillation strategies, thus, better defibrillators in the future.

The importance of TTI is further supported by a recent meta-analysis, concluding that skeletal muscles shunt away 82% of the electrical current while lung tissue shunts away 14% of the heart so that only 4% of the total level of electrical current reaches the heart [7]. This, besides raising some clinical questions, reinforces the need to gain a better understanding and insight into the factors that influence the level of TTI, hence the extent of electric current flow.

1.3 Definition and background of transthoracic impedance

The history of electrical defibrillation dates back to 1956, when a patient was successfully treated for ventricular fibrillation. A few years later, the delivery of an electric shock proved to be effective in atrial fibrillation and atrial flutter [8, 9].

Several factors have been investigated to make defibrillation therapy more effective, highlighting the paramount importance of the current application and the current delivery distribution [10]. Effective defibrillation is based on the delivery of an electrical shock to a critical amount of myocardial cells, which is determined by the flow of electrical current that is influenced by the shock energy modified according to the measured TTI. If the electrical current is too low, defibrillation will fail, so the objective should be to reduce the level of TTI as much as possible [11].

With the development of cardiac implantable devices, it has become possible to measure a variety of parameters, enabling healthcare specialists to provide telemedical treatment and monitoring. One of these parameters is the monitoring of the intrathoracic impedance in a special setup of implantable cardioverter defibrillators (ICDs) to monitor fluid overload in chronic heart failure patients. A recent meta-analysis has shown that reduced intrathoracic impedance is a significant risk factor for developing both atrial and ventricular arrhythmias [12]. However, in the present chapter, we focus on the factors affecting transthoracic impedance and do not address intrathoracic impedance because of the different measurement characteristics.

The factors that influence TTI can be divided into two subgroups, modifiable (extrinsic) and nonmodifiable (intrinsic) factors. Although the latter are not alterable, knowledge of them allows us to approximate the value of a TTI more accurately.

1.4 Methodology of transthoracic impedance measurements

The available datasets involving TTI measurements are derived mainly from implantable defibrillator devices and external defibrillators in the setting of electrophysiological conditions requiring the delivery of an electric shock to patients. The other technique is high-frequency impedance estimation. This is a built-in feature of all modern defibrillator devices, estimating what the current TTI value might be according to the so-called test-pulse method by delivering a minimum current electrical pulse.

2. Factors influencing transthoracic impedance

2.1 Paddle force, contact pressure

Several studies have examined the influence of electrode contact on the TTI, highlighting an inverse relation between electrode pressure and TTI [13–18]. When holding conventional, hand-held defibrillator paddles, by increasing the pressure force, the electrical contact surface at the electrode-skin contact level increases, while the air volume in the lungs may decrease [15]. The optimal paddle force is different for adults and children: 8 kilogram-force (kgf) for adults, 5 kgf for children, and 3 kgf for infants [13, 14].

Since 2020, the ERC guidelines have recommended the use of self-adhesive defibrillation pads instead of defibrillation paddles to improve defibrillation performance and increase the safety of the providers [19]. Although the importance of paddle force has been marginalized by the widespread use of defibrillation pads, studies indicate that the force applied to self-adhesive defibrillation pads may as well contribute to reduced TTI [17, 18, 20].

In addition to the absolute force applied, the size of the defibrillator electrode is also important, as it is a key element in the distribution of the pressure. This may be especially important in the case of defibrillating infants and children weighing less than 10 kg [7].

2.2 Pad/paddle placement

Human studies have failed to prove the role of the pad position as a determinant of Return of spontaneous circulation (ROSC) in the setting of ventricular tachycardias [19]. According to the ILCOR 2020 systematic review, trans-myocardial electrical flow is highest when the fibrillating myocardial area is located between the defibrillator electrodes. This indicates that the optimal position of the electrodes is the region located close to the left ventricle in cases of ventricular arrhythmia. Where feasible, anterolateral (sternal-apical) positioning is recommended; however, anteroposterior, bi-axillary, and right posterior-apical positionings are also acceptable. In large-breasted individuals, the electrode may be shifted to the lateral or inferior side, selecting the one closest to the optimal placement if possible [19, 21]. Deakin et al. found that the use of the apical defibrillation paddle in a longitudinal orientation resulted in a significantly lower TTI compared to the transverse placement during shocks in cardioversion [22].

2.3 Repeated shocks

The change in TTI during multiple shocks is also a topic of debate [23]. In their study, Deakin et al. conducted electrical cardioversion on 58 patients. TTI significantly decreased with each consecutive shock, initially averaging 92.2 Ohms, while for patients receiving five shocks, the average was 85.0 Ohms [24]. Similarly, Fumagalli and colleagues found a significant difference in TTI, which decreased by 6.2% after 2 or more shocks from the starting value [25]. However, Walker and colleagues analyzed data from 863 out-of-hospital cardiac arrest patients treated with AED shocks for ventricular fibrillation and found no significant change in TTI between consecutive shocks. In the study, they examined both the high-frequency impedance and the shock impedance; all patients were initially administered 200 J for their first shocks, with the second shocks being either 200 J or 300 J, using preprogrammed AEDs by the local protocols [26]. Niemann and colleagues also found similar results in their animal model, as TTI did not change significantly in animals receiving 4 or more shocks compared to the first shock to eliminate ventricular fibrillation [27].

2.4 Hypothermia

The beneficial role of induced hypothermia (HT) is still a widely debated issue, mainly as a measure to protect the heart and brain after cardiac arrest following resuscitation. According to Rhee and colleagues, severe HT enhanced the success of transthoracic defibrillation in a swine model. After inducing ventricular fibrillation for 30 s, the pigs were defibrillated using biphasic waveform at various energies in both normothermic and HT conditions. Results showed that severe HT (30°C) led to a higher success rate in terminating ventricular fibrillation compared to normothermia, even though impedance increased and current decreased during HT. No significant differences were found between normothermia and HT in the other groups [28]. Similarly, the moderate HT (33°C) group showed a significant increase in first-shock success, with a trend toward improvement in the severe HT group in another swine model [29]. The rise in defibrillation success despite the increased TTI in hypothermic conditions suggests that other factors besides current delivery may contribute to improved shock success.

2.5 Respiration phase

Sirna and colleagues observed 28 patients who underwent elective cardioversion and were monitored for 48 h after shock delivery and compared them with 10 control subjects who did not receive a shock. TTI was 9% lower at end-expiration compared to end-inspiration [15]. Kim and colleagues also confirmed that impedance seems to be sensitive to changes in lung volume and body position [30]. According to a study published in 2004, TTI drops as thoracic volume decreases, but this only accounts for a maximum of 16% of the total TTI reduction [31]. Deakin and colleagues also observed that TTI increased linearly with increasing positive end-expiratory pressure [32]. Furthermore, in another study, they examined 10 healthy people while they breathed different respiratory gas mixtures and concluded that TTI is unlikely to be affected by different breathing gases during defibrillation [33].

2.6 Coupling agent

The proper alignment and connection of electrodes to the skin are vital for achieving accurate TTI measurements. Sirna et al. found that using a salt-free adhesive gel (ultrasound gel) led to a 20% higher TTI compared to a salt-containing gel (Redux paste). When no adhesive was used, TTI was significantly higher than the control [15]. In a study, 80 patients were examined and received 267 shocks using self-adhesive electrode paddles. The researchers compared the effectiveness of these pads to traditional manual electrode paddles. The transthoracic impedance during defibrillation did not significantly differ between the self-adhesive pads and manual pads (75 ± 21 Ohm vs. 67 ± 36 Ohm). The initial shock success rate of 64% for ventricular fibrillation of self-adhesive pads using 150–200 J shock energy was found to be comparably good [34] to the defibrillation rates achieved in a large prospective study that achieved successful first shock in 61% of the total OHCA patients, delivering 175 J shock energy by defibrillation paddles [35]. Thus, self-adhesive pads were found to be effective for both defibrillation and cardioversion [34]. However, Dodd and colleagues found that using manual paddles resulted in lower TTI than using self-adhesive paddles in both the anterior-anterior and anterior-posterior positions [36]. This may be due to the pressure set on the paddles and body by defibrillation providers.

2.7 Age

The relationship between age and TTI is not well understood, and there is a lack of agreement among experts. Several studies have reported that TTI values are higher in older adults. This can be attributed to a variety of factors, including altered body posture as a result of musculoskeletal diseases associated with aging and decreased lung function [7, 37]. However, in a study by Fumagalli and colleagues, there was no correlation between age and chest impedance. This discrepancy may be explained by their study population being restricted to a narrow age range, with 75% of patients being around 70 years old [38]. Additionally, there was a high prevalence of chronic heart failure in the patient population, which is associated with lower chest impedance. Seung-Young Roh and colleagues performed a total of 683 direct current cardioversions in 466 patients with atrial tachyarrhythmias. In their study, they found that age did not affect TTI [39].

2.8 Gender

In a meta-analysis, Heyer and colleagues obtained contradictory results regarding the relationship between TTI and gender and found no clear trend. Body fat increases with age, to a greater extent, in women than in men [7]. From this, one might conclude that chest electrical impedance is higher in women; however, many other factors also differ between the two sexes, which makes the picture more nuanced. For example, chest hair also affects TTI. It has been shown that after shaving, chest impedance decreases significantly [40, 41]. In the 2020 ILCOR overview paper, the authors conclude that the removal of chest hair before electrode placement may be considered if it does not delay the shock delivery [42]. Overall, it can be said that factors that affect TTI, such as the amount of subcutaneous fat, or hair, and breast size, also show a high degree of variability within gender and that knowledge of these factors together would be necessary to tailor the delivered shock energy level to the individual.

2.9 Body mass index (BMI)

The results of the studies suggest that as BMI increases, chest impedance also increases [22, 38, 39, 43, 44]. The exact mechanism behind this is currently unknown. It is believed that increased amounts of fat tissue may lead to higher chest impedance values. Body composition measurement methods (InBody) also utilize this characteristic in their measurements [45].

2.10 Hemoglobin concentration

Studies have shown a connection between hemoglobin concentration and the electrical properties of blood [46]. Plasma is believed to be the conductive element of blood, with red blood cells interfering with current flow and increasing blood viscosity [47]. The microvascular tree itself alone acts as an electrical insulator due to the presence of endothelial and red blood cells along the capillary wall [48].

Studies have shown a correlation between hemoglobin oxygen saturation and TTI [25, 38]. According to one study, a $1.9 \pm 0.6\ \Omega$ increase in TTI with higher Hb concentration is related to the electrical properties of blood and the insulating layers around capillaries [38]. Another study found a $0.2 \pm 0.1\ \Omega$ increase in TTI with higher Hb O2 saturation, partially attributed to Chronic Obstructive Pulmonary Disease symptoms [25]. An animal study observed that hypoxia can affect TTI by changing cytoplasmic resistance and intercellular impedance [49]. Higher Hb O2 saturation results in a small increase in TTI, with clinical significance dependent on other pathological symptoms.

2.11 Presence of chronic heart failure

In chronic heart failure, transthoracic impedance also changes in parallel with the symptoms of heart failure, such as pulmonary congestion, decreasing the TTI value. Research has found that a decrease in TTI or intrathoracic impedance, as measured by Cardiac resynchronization therapy (CRT) and ICD devices, is linked to the severity of heart failure and the patient's prognosis [38, 50–52]. Measuring TTI can aid in predicting the severity of heart failure and the patient's prognosis, as well as assessing the effectiveness of the treatment (**Table 1**).

Influencing factor	Chapter section	Change of transthoracic impedance
Electrode pressure	2.1.	Decreases with pressure
Electrode size	2.1.	Decreases with electrode size
Electrode position	2.2.	Decreases in anteroposterior position
Repeated shocks	2.3.	Decreases with multiple shocks
Respiration and lung volume	2.5.	Increases with lung volume
Coupling agent	2.6.	Decreases for good coupling
Age	2.7.	Increases with age
Body size, Body Mass Index (BMI)	2.9.	Increases with body dimensions
Hemoglobin saturation	2.10.	Increases with Hemoglobin O2 saturation

Chapter sections: 2.1. Paddle force, contact pressure, 2.2. Pad/paddle placement, 2.3. Repeated shocks, 2.4. Hypothermia, 2.5. Respiration phase, 2.6. Coupling agent, 2.7. Age, 2.8. Gender, 2.9. Body mass index (BMI), 2.10. Hemoglobin concentration.

Table 1.
Influencing factors of TTI supported by a recent meta-analysis [7].

3. Conclusion

Defibrillators are one of the most important devices that can potentially save a person's life in emergency medical situations of SCD or AF by restoring normal heart rhythm. The TTI plays a key role in determining the current flow during defibrillation and should be monitored and used for current modulation, to improve the success and safety of the procedure. In this chapter, we have analyzed and discussed the most important factors that can affect TTI and, thus defibrillation success.

Conflict of interest

The authors declare no conflict of interest.

Acronyms and abbreviations

AF	atrial fibrillation
CRT	cardiac resynchronization therapy
DF	defibrillation
ECV	electrical cardioversion
HT	hypothermia
ICD	implantable cardioverter defibrillator
kgf	kilogram-force
OHCA	out-of-hospital cardiac arrest
ROSC	return of spontaneous circulation
SCD	sudden cardiac death
TTI	transthoracic impedance
VT	ventricular tachycardia
VF	ventricular fibrillation

Author details

Adam Pal-Jakab, Bettina Nagy, Boldizsar Kiss and Endre Zima*
Department of Cardiology, Semmelweis University Heart and Vascular Centre, Budapest, Hungary

*Address all correspondence to: zima.endre@med.semmelweis-univ.hu

IntechOpen

© 2023 The Author(s). Licensee IntechOpen. This chapter is distributed under the terms of the Creative Commons Attribution License (http://creativecommons.org/licenses/by/3.0), which permits unrestricted use, distribution, and reproduction in any medium, provided the original work is properly cited.

References

[1] Grasner JT, Wnent J, Herlitz J, Perkins GD, Lefering R, Tjelmeland I, et al. Survival after out-of-hospital cardiac arrest in Europe - results of the EuReCa TWO study. Resuscitation. 2020;**148**:218-226

[2] Empana J-P, Lerner I, Valentin E, Folke F, Böttiger B, Gislason G, et al. Incidence of sudden cardiac death in the European Union. Journal of the American College of Cardiology. 2022;**79**(18):1818-1827

[3] Kong MH, Fonarow GC, Peterson ED, Curtis AB, Hernandez AF, Sanders GD, et al. Systematic review of the incidence of sudden cardiac death in the United States. Journal of the American College of Cardiology. 2011;**57**(7):794-801

[4] Stecker EC, Reinier K, Marijon E, Narayanan K, Teodorescu C, Uy-Evanado A, et al. Public health burden of sudden cardiac death in the United States. Circulation. Arrhythmia and Electrophysiology. 2014;**7**(2):212-217

[5] Priori SG, Blomstrom-Lundqvist C, Mazzanti A, Blom N, Borggrefe M, Camm J, et al. 2015 ESC guidelines for the management of patients with ventricular arrhythmias and the prevention of sudden cardiac death: The task force for the Management of Patients with ventricular arrhythmias and the prevention of sudden cardiac death of the European Society of Cardiology (ESC). Endorsed by: Association for European Paediatric and Congenital Cardiology (AEPC). European Heart Journal. 2015;**36**(41):2793-2867

[6] Hindricks G, Potpara T, Dagres N, Arbelo E, Bax JJ, Blomström-Lundqvist C, et al. 2020 ESC guidelines for the diagnosis and management of atrial fibrillation developed in collaboration with the European Association for Cardio-Thoracic Surgery (EACTS): The Task Force for the diagnosis and management of atrial fibrillation of the European Society of Cardiology (ESC) developed with the special contribution of the European Heart Rhythm Association (EHRA) of the ESC. European Heart Journal. 2020;**42**(5):373-498

[7] Heyer Y, Baumgartner D, Baumgartner C. A systematic review of the transthoracic impedance during cardiac defibrillation. Sensors. 2022;**22**(7):2808

[8] Lown B, Amarasingham R, Neuman J. New method for terminating cardiac arrhythmias. Use of synchronized capacitor discharge. Jama. 1962;**182**:548-555

[9] Lown B. Electrical reversion of cardiac arrhythmias. British Heart Journal. 1967;**29**(4):469-489

[10] KenKnight BH, Eyüboğlu BM, Ideker RE. Impedance to defibrillation countershock: Does an optimal impedance exist? Pacing and Clinical Electrophysiology. 1995;**18**(11):2068-2087

[11] Sado DM, Deakin CD. How good is your defibrillation technique? Journal of the Royal Society of Medicine. 2005;**98**(1):3-6

[12] Abubakar H, Osman M, Akintoye E, Subahi A, Osman K, Abidov A. Intra-thoracic impedance and the onset of atrial and ventricular tachyarrhythmias: A meta-analysis. International Journal of Cardiology. 2018;**258**:144-150

[13] Deakin CD, Sado DM, Petley GW, Clewlow F. Determining the optimal

paddle force for external defibrillation. The American Journal of Cardiology. 2002;**90**(7):812-813

[14] Deakin CD, Bennetts SH, Petley GW, Clewlow F. What is the optimal paddle force during paediatric external defibrillation? Resuscitation. 2003;**59**(1):83-88

[15] Sirna SJ, Ferguson DW, Charbonnier F, Kerber RE. Factors affecting transthoracic impedance during electrical cardioversion. The American Journal of Cardiology. 1988;**62**(16):1048-1052

[16] Kerber RE, Grayzel J, Hoyt R, Marcus M, Kennedy J. Transthoracic resistance in human defibrillation. Influence of body weight, chest size, serial shocks, paddle size and paddle contact pressure. Circulation. 1981;**63**(3):676-682

[17] Ramirez FD, Fiset SL, Cleland MJ, Zakutney TJ, Nery PB, Nair GM, et al. Effect of applying force to self-adhesive electrodes on transthoracic impedance: Implications for electrical cardioversion. Pacing and Clinical Electrophysiology. 2016;**39**(10):1141-1147

[18] Persse DE, Dzwonczyk R, Brown CG. Effect of application of force to self-adhesive defibrillator pads on transthoracic electrical impedance and countershock success. Annals of Emergency Medicine. 1999;**34**(2):129-133

[19] Soar J, Böttiger BW, Carli P, Couper K, Deakin CD, Djärv T, et al. European resuscitation council guidelines 2021: Adult advanced life support. Resuscitation. 2021;**161**:115-151

[20] Cohen TJ, Ibrahim B, Denier D, Haji A, Quan W. Active compression cardioversion for refractory atrial fibrillation. The American Journal of Cardiology. 1997;**80**(3):354-355

[21] Olasveengen TM, Mancini ME, Perkins GD, Avis S, Brooks S, Castrén M, et al. Adult basic life support: International consensus on cardiopulmonary resuscitation and emergency cardiovascular care science with treatment recommendations. Resuscitation. 2020;**156**:A35-a79

[22] Deakin CD, Sado DM, Petley GW, Clewlow F. Is the orientation of the apical defibrillation paddle of importance during manual external defibrillation? Resuscitation. 2003;**56**(1):15-18

[23] Kerber RE, Kouba C, Martins J, Kelly K, Low R, Hoyt R, et al. Advance prediction of transthoracic impedance in human defibrillation and cardioversion: Importance of impedance in determining the success of low-energy shocks. Circulation. 1984;**70**(2):303-308

[24] Deakin CD, Ambler JJ, Shaw S. Changes in transthoracic impedance during sequential biphasic defibrillation. Resuscitation. 2008;**78**(2):141-145

[25] Fumagalli S, Tarantini F, Caldi F, Makhanian Y, Padeletti M, Boncinelli L, et al. Multiple shocks affect thoracic electrical impedance during external cardioversion of atrial fibrillation. Pacing and Clinical Electrophysiology. 2009;**32**(3):371-377

[26] Walker RG, Koster RW, Sun C, Moffat G, Barger J, Dodson PP, et al. Defibrillation probability and impedance change between shocks during resuscitation from out-of-hospital cardiac arrest. Resuscitation 2009;**80**(7):773-7

[27] Niemann JT, Garner D, Lewis RJ. Transthoracic impedance does not decrease with rapidly repeated countershocks in a swine cardiac arrest model. Resuscitation. 2003;**56**(1):91-95

[28] Rhee BJ, Zhang Y, Boddicker KA, Davies LR, Kerber RE. Effect of hypothermia on transthoracic defibrillation in a swine model. Resuscitation. 2005;**65**(1):79-85

[29] Boddicker KA, Zhang Y, Zimmerman MB, Davies LR, Kerber RE. Hypothermia improves defibrillation success and resuscitation outcomes from ventricular fibrillation. Circulation. 2005;**111**(24):3195-3201

[30] Kim CH, Fuglestad MA, Richert ML, Shen WK, Johnson BD. Influence of lung volume, fluid and capillary recruitment during positional changes and exercise on thoracic impedance in heart failure. Respiratory Physiology & Neurobiology. 2014;**202**:75-81

[31] Deakin CD, Sado DM, Petley GW, Clewlow F. Differential contribution of skin impedance and thoracic volume to transthoracic impedance during external defibrillation. Resuscitation. 2004;**60**(2):171-174

[32] Deakin CD, McLaren RM, Petley GW, Clewlow F, Dalrymple-Hay MJ. Effects of positive end-expiratory pressure on transthoracic impedance—Implications for defibrillation. Resuscitation. 1998;**37**(1):9-12

[33] Deakin CD, McLaren RM, Pack LS, Petley GW, Clewlow F, Dalrymple-Hay MJ. Effects of respiratory gas composition on transthoracic impedance. Resuscitation. 1998;**38**(3):193-195

[34] Kerber RE, Martins JB, Kelly KJ, Ferguson DW, Kouba C, Jensen SR, et al. Self-adhesive preapplied electrode pads for defibrillation and cardioversion. Journal of the American College of Cardiology. 1984;**3**(3):815-820

[35] Weaver WD, Cobb LA, Copass MK, Hallstrom AP. Ventricular defibrillation—A comparative trial using 175-J and 320-J shocks. The New England Journal of Medicine. 1982;**307**(18):1101-1106

[36] Dodd TE, Deakin CD, Petley GW, Clewlow F. External defibrillation in the left lateral position—A comparison of manual paddles with self-adhesive pads. Resuscitation. 2004;**63**(3):283-286

[37] Garcia LA, Kerber RE. Transthoracic defibrillation: Does electrode adhesive pad position alter transthoracic impedance? Resuscitation. 1998;**37**(3):139-143

[38] Fumagalli S, Boni N, Padeletti M, Gori F, Boncinelli L, Valoti P, et al. Determinants of thoracic electrical impedance in external electrical cardioversion of atrial fibrillation. The American Journal of Cardiology. 2006;**98**(1):82-87

[39] Roh S-Y, Ahn J, Lee K-N, Baek Y-S, Kim D-H, Lee D-I, et al. The impact of personal thoracic impedance on electrical cardioversion in patients with atrial arrhythmias. Medicina. 2021;**57**(6):618

[40] Sado DM, Deakin CD, Petley GW, Clewlow F. Comparison of the effects of removal of chest hair with not doing so before external defibrillation on transthoracic impedance. The American Journal of Cardiology. 2004;**93**(1):98-100

[41] Bissing JW, Kerber RE. Effect of shaving the chest of hirsute subjects on transthoracic impedance to self-adhesive defibrillation electrode pads. The American Journal of Cardiology. 2000;**86**(5):587-589 a10

[42] Olasveengen TM, Mancini ME, Perkins GD, Avis S, Brooks S, Castrén M, et al. Adult basic life support. Resuscitation. 2020;**156**:A35-A79

[43] Ogunnaike BO, Whitten CW, Minhajuddin A, Melikman E, Joshi GP, Moon TS, et al. Body mass index and outcomes of in-hospital ventricular tachycardia and ventricular fibrillation arrest. Resuscitation. 2016;**105**:156-160

[44] Voskoboinik A, Moskovitch J, Plunkett G, Bloom J, Wong G, Nalliah C, et al. Cardioversion of atrial fibrillation in obese patients: Results from the cardioversion-BMI randomized controlled trial. Journal of Cardiovascular Electrophysiology. 2019;**30**(2):155-161

[45] Lemos T, Gallagher D. Current body composition measurement techniques. Current Opinion in Endocrinology, Diabetes, and Obesity. 2017;**24**(5):310-314

[46] Ishihara T, Igarashi I, Kitano T, Shinzato T, Maeda K. Continuous hematocrit monitoring method in an extracorporeal circulation system and its application for automatic control of blood volume during artificial kidney treatment. Artificial Organs. 1993;**17**(8):708-716

[47] Hoetink AE, Faes TJ, Visser KR, Heethaar RM. On the flow dependency of the electrical conductivity of blood. IEEE Transactions on Biomedical Engineering. 2004;**51**(7):1251-1261

[48] Fleischhauer J, Lehmann L, Kléber AG. Electrical resistances of interstitial and microvascular space as determinants of the extracellular electrical field and velocity of propagation in ventricular myocardium. Circulation. 1995;**92**(3):587-594

[49] Wojtczak J. Contractures and increase in internal longitudianl resistance of cow ventricular muscle induced by hypoxia. Circulation Research. 1979;**44**(1):88-95

[50] Maines M, Catanzariti D, Cirrincione C, Valsecchi S, Comisso J, Vergara G. Intrathoracic impedance and pulmonary wedge pressure for the detection of heart failure deterioration. Europace. 2010;**12**(5):680-685

[51] Vollmann D, Nägele H, Schauerte P, Wiegand U, Butter C, Zanotto G, et al. Clinical utility of intrathoracic impedance monitoring to alert patients with an implanted device of deteriorating chronic heart failure. European Heart Journal. 2007;**28**(15):1835-1840

[52] Whellan DJ, Droogan CJ, Fitzpatrick J, Adams S, McCarey MM, Andrel J, et al. Change in intrathoracic impedance measures during acute decompensated heart failure admission: Results from the diagnostic data for discharge in heart failure patients (3D-HF) pilot study. Journal of Cardiac Failure. 2012;**18**(2):107-112